Balance Exercises for Seniors

Building Strength, Flexibility, and Stability with Effective Workouts

Table of Contents

Introduction

Aging is not for the faint of heart. When you think about the importance of being stable on your feet, it becomes evident that aging is not a path meant for those who lose their footing. If you've ever fallen, regardless of your age, you're well aware of how awkward and embarrassing it can be, especially if your stumble unfolds in front of an audience. Luckily, you might have emerged unscathed, experienced minor inconveniences like bruises, strains, or sprains, or perhaps encountered more severe injuries that hampered your daily activities, like broken or dislocated bones.

However, if you've managed to avoid falling, it's not yet time to boast. Why, you might ask? As you grow older, your muscles lose some of their strength, and your reflexes slow down. Unfortunately, this makes the risk of falling increase with each passing day. As you approach your 60s, 70s, 80s, and beyond, retaining strength and stability becomes essential for leading a vibrant and active life.

According to the Centers for Disease Control and Prevention, over 1 in 4 seniors fall every year and a staggering 3 million end up in hospitals due to fall-related injuries. However, here's the good news: you've landed in the right place. You won't become just another statistic. Falls are not accepted as a normal part of the aging process. Nevertheless, every year, millions of older adults lose their balance, slipping and falling and often incurring severe injury. The statistics provided by the Centers for Disease Control and Prevention (CDCP) shed light on the seriousness of the issue:

- A quarter of adults aged 65 and older experience a fall each year.

- If you've fallen once, your likelihood of falling again doubles.

- Emergency rooms nationwide treat over three million older adults for fall-related injuries, with 800,000 of those requiring hospitalization due to head or hip injuries resulting from their falls.

- One-fifth of falls result in serious injuries, such as head trauma or broken bones.

- Traumatic brain injuries are most frequently caused by falls.

- Shockingly, over 95 percent of hip fractures are the direct result of a fall (CDCP, 2019).

The balance exercises provided in this book can be a valuable resource for enhancing your strength and improving balance. However, please do recognize that everyone's needs and conditions are unique. So, before you start an exercise program, consulting a qualified physical therapist or a physician is essential, especially if the exercise routine seems challenging. This consultation is particularly crucial if you have recently undergone surgery related to arthritis, bunions, joint discomfort, or mobility issues.

Chapter 1: Understanding Balance

Slips and falls are the most common causes of injuries in senior citizens. Besides having decreased muscle strength, the root cause of falls in senior citizens is balance issues. When the body loses its ability to maintain balance partially or entirely, the chances of slips or falls increase. Balance exercises can be the secret weapon in your arsenal that mitigates issues with maintaining balance. Effectively practicing these exercises, especially in old age, keeps you going in life with rhythm, without fear of mobility limitations or balance issues.

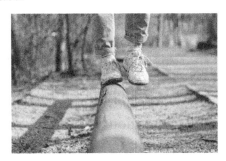

1. Balance exercises can be the secret weapon in your arsenal that mitigates issues with maintaining balance. Source: https://pixabay.com/photos/balance-bar-shoes-feet-person-6157258/

Incorporating balance exercises is crucial for seniors because senior life should be fulfilling and independent. These exercises can prime anyone's body to perform at optimum levels and significantly help improve overall health. Here's why balance exercises and their myriad benefits are a must-do for seniors:

The Necessity of Balance Exercises for Seniors

Falls Prevention

With age, every metabolic process in the body decreases in efficiency. This gradual decrease in metabolism has effects throughout the body. The muscles weaken, and the mineral deposits in bones deplete, leading to reduced bone density.

Other factors like decreased appetite, reduced ability of intestines to absorb food, and a plethora of medical conditions also contribute to decreased mobility. Statistics from the World Health Organization revealed that falls are the second leading cause of accidental injury and death, especially among seniors. Balance exercises can prime the body, enhance stability, and reduce the likelihood of debilitating falls.

Staying Independent

When you lose balance, it affects your independence. Increasing balance issues may make performing simple mobility tasks or house chores difficult. In these circumstances, performing a task can result in falls, injuries, or fractures that will take time to heal and recover. Fortifying equilibrium with balance exercises will ensure you can do whatever you want, the way you like.

Enhanced Mobility

With balance exercises, you will not only improve steadiness but also improve mobility. This improved mobility and balance can let you enjoy outdoor activities, take leisure walks at your favorite park, or have an outdoor adventure with your grandchildren.

The Benefits of Regular Balance Exercises for Seniors

Improved Physical Health

Balance exercises strengthen the core muscles and help correct posture, leading to more stability when done correctly. The increased muscle tone significantly aids in supporting already weak bones and joints and reduces the risk of conditions like osteoarthritis (inflammation of bones and joints).

Mental Well-Being

Like decreased metabolism and muscle strength, cognitive function declines with age. Balance exercises provide the right amount of cognitive stimulation, ultimately sharpening cognitive function. This increased ability to concentrate and keep the head clear also prevents the development of neurological conditions like dementia (loss of cognitive functioning affecting remembering, thinking, and reasoning).

Confidence Boost

These exercises are a natural confidence booster, fostering a sense of achievement. This motivation can make you keep going to stay active and focus on your overall well-being.

Social Engagement

Besides allowing you to go out and be yourself on your terms, balance exercises are excellent for fostering social connections and combating loneliness. You can perform these exercises with your partner or a group of friends, which will benefit everyone involved and develop stronger bonds.

Better Quality of Life

These physical and mental benefits fostered by regular balance exercises significantly improve quality of life in the long run. Seniors capable of maintaining balance are more likely to enjoy their golden years.

Balance exercises aren't just another entry on your fitness checklist. It's a well-defined path that enables you to empower your body and defy age-related limitations. You'll gain physical strength, boost mental resilience, and the freedom to embrace every moment.

The Science of Balance

Balancing in humans is maintained through complex interaction and coordination of the body, senses, and brain. While it can take much time and reading to understand complex processes and interactions that maintain balance in the human body, the information presented here is simple enough to familiarize you with these processes.

The Sensory Systems

The human body uses its sensory systems of hearing, vision, and movement to maintain balance. The process starts with sensory input from the following three systems.

Vestibular System

Located in the inner ear, it contributes majorly to maintaining balance. This system has three semicircular and hollow canal-like structures containing hair cells, fluid, and sac-like otolith organs that respond to gravitational forces. When the head moves or the body changes position, all structures in the vestibular system pick up the changes occurring with head position and motion. These detected changes are converted into signals and sent to the brain, providing crucial information about the orientation and motion of the body.

Visual System

The eyes assist in visualizing objects, noting their position, and scanning the surroundings to know about your position relative to the surroundings. These visual cues are also signaled to the brain, further assisting in maintaining balance.

Proprioceptive System

The proprioceptive system receptors are embedded in muscles, joints, and tendons. These receptors gather information regarding joint positions, muscle tension, and the changes in muscle length during their contraction and relaxation. This sensory information is sent to the brain, informing about the limb position and the effort needed to maintain balance.

The Brain's Role

The brain processes all the sensory information from the three primary sensory systems and orchestrates an appropriate response. The three major parts of the brain aiding in initiating the required response are:

Brainstem

The brainstem receives signals from the vestibular system and processes information about the head's position and movement. Then, it relays this information to other brain parts, including the cerebellum and the cerebral cortex.

Cerebellum

The cerebellum fine-tunes the motor control and coordination. Motor control is the human body's ability to coordinate and activate muscles to maintain posture. The cerebellum also receives sensory information from the proprioceptive system to further adjust to maintain balance.

Cerebral Cortex

The parietal and frontal lobes of the cerebral cortex are involved in processing higher-level balance information. It integrates sensory input from all three systems and helps you adapt to complex situations, like walking on uneven terrain or standing on one foot.

The Balance Control Loop

Maintaining balance is an ongoing process. It involves a continuous feedback loop, during which sensory input from all three systems streams into the brain, like a thermostat regulating room temperature—s. The brain processes this information, determining your current position and orientation.

Based on the brain's calculations, respective signals are sent to the required muscles to maintain balance and adjust position. During movement, the sensory system keeps monitoring the muscle movement, providing feedback to the brain, allowing it to fine-tune the signals and recalibrate balance accordingly.

Challenges to Balance

Balance is affected by several factors, including the following:

Age: As the human body ages, the sensitivity of the vestibular system decreases, and muscle strength diminishes, affecting balance.

Medical Conditions: Severe ear infections, ear disorders, diseases, brain-related conditions, and accidents affecting inner ear structures are common conditions impairing balance.

Environmental Factors: Situations like walking on uneven surfaces and areas with poor lighting can affect your balance.

Medications: Prolonged intake of medicines for certain diseases and medical conditions can affect balance and coordination.

Training and Adaptation

Although several factors affect balance, performing regular balance exercises and training can significantly improve muscle strength and posture. This regular practice enhances the brain's communication with sensory systems, further improving balance.

It's a remarkable feat of biological engineering, allowing you to navigate the world with grace and poise. Understanding the science behind balance can help you appreciate the intricate mechanisms that keep you on your feet. It underscores the importance of maintaining and improving this vital skill throughout life.

Common Balance Issues in Seniors

Balance issues in seniors can arise from various factors, and understanding these common problems is crucial for effective prevention and management. Here's a detailed explanation of some of the most common balance issues.

Muscle Weakness

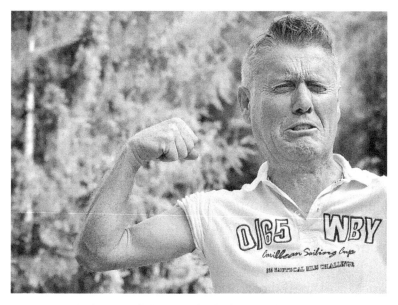

2. *Sarcopenia is a condition in which the muscles lose their strength and become weak. Source: https://pixabay.com/photos/cartoon-man-weak-effort-no-muscles-812270/*

Besides muscle wasting (muscles lose their tone and strength), elderly people can develop sarcopenia, a condition in which the muscles lose their strength and become weak, making it difficult to maintain balance. Core and leg muscles are affected the most in sarcopenia. Once the condition develops, you may face difficulty switching between postures like standing, walking, or changing body positions.

Reduced Proprioception

Another age-related balance issue is reduced proprioception. It becomes difficult to perceive the position of body parts as the sensors in the muscles, tendons, and joints become less receptive. Reduced proprioception makes it extremely difficult to adjust posture or better control core muscles to reduce the risk of falls.

Changes in Vision

Changes in peripheral vision, decreased visual acuity, and faulty depth perception are some vision-related issues diminishing the ability to detect potential environmental hazards. Impaired vision makes it harder to navigate obstacles and maintain stability.

Vestibular System Changes

The vestibular system in the inner ear may undergo age-related changes, leading to decreased sensitivity of the structures involved in maintaining balance. This can affect detecting head movements and maintaining balance. Vestibular dysfunction can result in dizziness, vertigo, balance, and spatial orientation difficulties.

Medications

Many seniors take multiple medications for various health conditions. Some medications, particularly those affecting the central nervous system, can have side effects like dizziness or impaired coordination. These side effects increase seniors' risk of falls and balance problems, especially when taking multiple medications.

Neuropathy

Neuropathy refers to damage or dysfunction of nerves, which occur due to various causes, including diabetes, chemotherapy, or other medical conditions. Neuropathy can result in numbness, tingling, or loss of sensation in the feet and legs, making it challenging to detect uneven surfaces and maintain balance.

Joint Problems

Arthritis and joint conditions are more common in older adults and can cause pain, stiffness, and reduced joint mobility. Joint pain and limited joint range of motion can affect the ability to adjust posture and move smoothly, leading to balance issues.

Cognitive Decline

Cognitive decline due to conditions like dementia, Alzheimer's, Parkinson's, etc., decreases the ability to process sensory information, make decisions, and react quickly. Cognitive impairment leads to confusion, disorientation, and poor judgment, increasing the risk of falls and balance-related accidents.

Fear of Falling

After experiencing a fall due to loss of balance, some seniors develop a fear of falling, which can lead to reduced physical activity and further muscle weakness. A fear of falling can become a self-fulfilling prophecy, as reduced physical activity leads to weaker muscles and decreased balance, perpetuating the cycle.

Environmental Factors

Seniors may encounter environmental hazards like slippery floors, inadequate lighting, or uneven surfaces in their homes or communities. These factors increase the risk of falls and contribute to balance issues in seniors, especially when combined with other physical or sensory challenges.

Orthostatic Hypotension

Orthostatic hypotension is a sudden drop in blood pressure when a person stands from a sitting or lying position. It can lead to dizziness and loss of balance. Seniors with orthostatic hypotension are at risk of falling when they stand up, especially if the condition is not properly managed.

Foot Problems

Foot conditions like bunions, hammer toes, and corns can affect foot alignment and alter weight distribution when standing and walking. Active foot issues can cause discomfort and increase instability, making it challenging to maintain balance while walking.

Dehydration

Dehydration is a common issue among seniors as they develop reduced thirst perception. It becomes difficult for them to recognize whether they are thirsty. Increased dehydration results in dizziness and weakness, and severe cases can cause cognitive impairment. These problems rooted in dehydration significantly increase the risk of falls.

Stroke or Brain Injury Sequelae

Seniors who have experienced a stroke or traumatic brain injury may develop residual effects, such as weakness, paralysis, or changes in coordination. The physical impairments resulting from stroke or brain injury can significantly make maintaining balance and performing daily activities challenging.

Neurological Disorders

Neurological conditions like multiple sclerosis and peripheral neuropathy affect nerve function and coordination. These disorders result in muscle stiffness, tremors, and impaired motor skills, contributing to balance problems.

Altered Gait Patterns

Seniors develop altered gait patterns, such as shuffling steps or a wide-based gait. due to various factors like pain, joint stiffness, or neurological conditions Altered gait patterns can disrupt the normal biomechanics of walking and increase the risk of falls.

Ear Disorders

Ear disorders like Ménière's disease or benign paroxysmal positional vertigo (BPPV) can cause dizziness and balance disturbances. Seniors with ear disorders may experience sudden episodes of vertigo or unsteadiness, making it challenging to maintain balance.

Lack of Physical Activity

A sedentary lifestyle leads to muscle weakness, decreased joint flexibility, and reduced cardiovascular fitness, impacting balance. Seniors who do not engage in regular physical activity will find it more challenging to maintain balance and overall physical health.

Seniors could experience a combination of these factors, making it even more crucial to address balance issues comprehensively. Balance exercises, regular medical check-ups, and appropriate lifestyle modifications significantly improve seniors' balance, enhancing their overall well-being and reducing the risk of falls and related injuries.

Understanding these common balance issues and identifying them in a timely fashion is essential. Addressing these challenges through preventive measures, rehabilitation, and appropriate interventions significantly improves the quality of life and safety.

Assessing Your Balance

Whether you have a medical condition interfering with the body's ability to maintain balance or just old age, assessing the balance to identify the potential issue further and take the necessary steps to mitigate it is essential. Here are some things you can do to learn more about balance, making it easier to address the underlying causes.

Berg Balance Scale

This is a more comprehensive assessment performed by a healthcare professional. It involves a series of tasks, like sitting to standing, reaching, and maintaining balance on one leg. A score on the Berg Balance Scale provides a more detailed evaluation of your balance abilities.

Consulting a Healthcare Professional

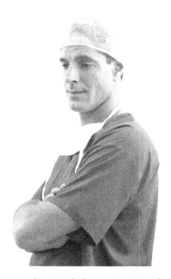

3. Consulting a healthcare provider or physical therapist is advisable if you have concerns about your balance. Source: https://pixabay.com/photos/isolated-doctor-dentist-dental-care-1188036/

Consulting a healthcare provider or physical therapist is advisable if you have concerns about your balance. They will conduct a thorough assessment, including a medical history review, physical examination, and specialized balance tests.

Use of Technology

Many mobility rehabilitation centers use tech to log the progress and tweak exercises according to the physical capabilities for maximum impact. Digital tools and apps are also available to assess balance. These tools and apps use accelerometers or other sensors to provide objective measurements. Contact a certified physiotherapist for advice on which tech to use and a balanced exercise plan tailored to your body's limitations.

Over many years, several tests to evaluate balance have been introduced to gain different insights regarding balance. Here are some popular balance tests you can check out.

Single Leg Balance Test

- Find a flat surface and ensure that there are no objects lying around.
- Perform this exercise near a tabletop or a window for extra support.
- Keep your arms at your sides or behind your back.
- Now, maintain balance for as long as possible.
- Record the time it takes until you lose balance, sway significantly, or need to put your foot down.

This test assesses your ability to balance on one leg, which is essential for activities like walking, climbing stairs, and getting out of a chair. It provides a simple measure of your lower body strength and stability. Balancing for at least 30 seconds on each leg is generally considered a good sign of lower body strength and balance.

Tandem Stand Test

- Stand with one foot directly in front of the other so that the heel of your front foot touches the toes of your back foot.

- Maintain this tandem stance for at least 30 seconds.

- Note any swaying, falling to the side, or needing to step out of the tandem position.

The tandem stand test evaluates your ability to balance on a narrow support base, which mimics challenging real-life situations like walking along a tightrope. It helps assess your proprioception and ankle stability, as maintaining this position requires fine motor control.

Romberg Test

- Stand with your feet close together, heels touching, and your arms at your sides.

- Close your eyes and try to maintain this position for 30 seconds.

- Note any swaying or significant imbalance.

The Romberg test challenges your balance without visual input, relying solely on your proprioceptive and vestibular systems. If you have difficulty maintaining balance with your eyes closed, it could indicate sensory input or proprioception issues.

Functional Reach Test

- Stand beside a wall with your arm extended horizontally, parallel to the floor.

- Without moving your feet, reach as far forward as you can without losing balance or taking a step.

- Measure the distance you reached.

The functional reach test assesses your dynamic balance and stability while reaching for objects. A shorter reach suggests a decreased ability to maintain balance when reaching, which is necessary for daily activities.

Timed up and Go Test

- Start by sitting in a sturdy chair with armrests.

- Place a marker or cone on the floor about 10 feet away.

- When ready, stand, walk to the marker, turn around, return to the chair, and sit down.

- Measure the time it takes to complete the task.

The Timed Up test assesses your mobility and ability to perform daily tasks transitioning from sitting to standing and walking. Longer times could indicate balance or mobility issues and an increased risk of falls.

These balance assessments can provide valuable insights into your balance capabilities and potential issues. Remember, individual results vary based on age, fitness, and health conditions. Suppose you have concerns about your balance or experience difficulties during these tests. In that case, consult a healthcare professional or physical therapist for a more comprehensive assessment and guidance on improving your balance. Maintaining balance is crucial for preventing falls and ensuring overall mobility and quality of life as you age.

Chapter 2: Getting Started

Taking the decision to radically change the quality of your life by embracing balancing exercise is one you will not regret. With age comes numerous ailments that can be lingering and are life-altering. Physical activity can help with many of these age-related illnesses like diabetes, cardiovascular problems, and strokes. Regular exercise has been shown to slow the onset rate of dementia. In addition to the physical benefits of exercising, working out can aid with mental health, too. Jumping head first into physical activity with consideration for your safety can relieve stress and promote a sense of achievement in your later years.

There are few feelings better than a good stretch. Taking a deep breath in, pulling your muscles to their limit, and then releasing the tension with a sigh brings an instant relaxing satisfaction. Stretching does not need to be viewed as a chore but can be a great hobby and a way to clear your mind from the worries of the day. The book's numerous stretches target your whole body and give you enough options to vary your daily workout so you never get bored. Many people are keen to get started with exercise but look past the benefits that simple stretches unlock. The way your body feels after a thorough stretch routine leaves you rejuvenated and ready to face the day's challenges.

One often overlooked issue that elderly people experience is the fear of falling. Falls can be terrifying as you adjust to the altered sense of equilibrium and age-related muscle and joint pain. It causes many to become inactive due to having previously fallen or experiencing close calls. Balance exercise can do restorative work to help you regain much of your independence and freedom of movement. Age does not have to be a hindrance to full emergence in the beauty of life. Balance exercises can reawaken so much that is missed out on with immobility and inactivity.

The start of a journey is always the most difficult. You are now establishing a new routine to regain your bodily wealth and enjoy the body you live in. This chapter will guide you on how to correctly and safely begin working on your balance with workouts that engage your entire body. Balance is a dynamic biological process that uses your arms, legs, and core to increase your health from top to bottom as every muscle works to your benefit. A gradual climb into the world of balancing exercise will give you renewed vitality.

Safety Precautions

As people age, the body answers back for all the years of misuse. You cannot exert the same force on yourself that you once did, and you take a lot longer to recover from injuries. What could have been quickly brushed off in your twenties could result in weeks in bed in your sixties or seventies. Safety becomes a crucial concern when exercising for the elderly. The aim of balance exercise is to increase your overall health and prevent falling. If you get injured while training or fall while exercising, the workout's purpose is defeated. A safe foundation must be laid before any activity.

With simple guidance, you can safely exercise and extract all the advantages from your workout routine. Embracing safety protocols maximizes your sessions by ensuring you are helped and not harmed to enjoy your prime elderly years wholeheartedly. Before you start a new exercise routine, it is essential to visit your doctor. Knowing the condition of your body and what is medically advised will shape the exercises you can do. It is easy to become overzealous and tumble into self-destruction. Therefore, consulting a medical professional takes the blinkers off of what is happening inside you so that you can proceed with the due caution required.

Set a comfortable pace, and do not feel the need to overexert yourself. Consistently doing a little goes a long way. When you do too much, your schedule can become erratic because you will need extra time to recover. The stop-and-start system coupled with the constant injury caused by pushing your limits is a breeding ground for quitting. Gradually getting a rhythm going is a long-term strategy that works. You can increase the intensity little by little when you feel you can do more, but not rush anything. As long as you put in the work daily, results will come. Trying to speed up the process will only invite excessive injuries. There is also a risk of sustaining an injury that keeps you from exercising permanently.

Warming up and cooling down cannot be taken for granted. Collagen is a protein responsible in part for elasticity in your skin and joints. Older people lose collagen over time, hence, the elderly are wrinkled. However, your skin is not the only part of your body affected by collagen loss because your joints and muscles are also no longer as flexible. Therefore, warming up and cooling down is increasingly essential as you age. Your body is not at the level it once was. Treating yourself the same way you did twenty years ago is unfair to your potential progress, and you will most likely hit a barrier if you skip the essential steps of warming up and cooling down.

Caring for your body is not only about exercise. You must listen to what your muscles and joints tell you, especially as you age. Your body does not communicate in words but shouts out with pain and discomfort signals. Stretches are meant to be uncomfortable but not meant to hurt. If you feel you are experiencing excessive pain when completing a stretch, it may not be the right exercise for you. Instead, attempt a gentler version of the stretch instead of pushing your body beyond its limits. Being overly ambitious and getting injured defeats the purpose of stretching: to increase your flexibility and reduce pain so you can have a higher quality of life.

Warming up prepares you for physical activity. Your muscles and essential organs like your lungs and heart are used when you exercise. Warm-up exercises allow the blood to flow to the needed areas to prepare your muscles and organs for an increase in activity. This preparation reduces the risk of injury and helps promote a faster recovery. Cooling down after working out allows your body to readjust to a less intense state. Failing to cool down can result in muscle soreness, stiffness, dizziness, nausea, and fainting. The increased blood flow in your muscles should be gradually released into your system to smooth the transition between being active and resting.

Avoid working out by yourself. Nobody plans on getting injured, but you must prepare for all possibilities. Having a capable partner around in case of emergencies is a decision you will not regret. You may require assistance with various exercises or need encouragement, and having someone present makes the process more enjoyable and less lonely.

Even if you feel you are more than capable of doing the balancing work yourself, having an unnecessary workout partner is better than suddenly finding yourself needing one and having nobody around. If your partner is knowledgeable, they will guide your workouts and ensure that you get the best results. Walking a fitness and wellness path can be difficult, but with someone assisting you along the way, you can remain steadfast in your health goals.

Hydration is one of the primary pillars of safe workout sessions. You will sweat and lose a lot of liquid during exercises, so you must make sure to replace the fluid you lose. Always have a water bottle by your side and drink whenever you feel thirsty. Fueling your body is central to safety, so eating a healthy diet prevents injury and speeds up recovery. Your body is mostly water, so the importance of the life-giving liquid cannot be understated.

The conditions you work in are central to your safety. Extreme temperatures affect your body's functions, so do not work out in extreme cold or heat. Your temperature should be maintained at a comfortable level. The air quality and ventilation of the space must be considered because breathing affects performance. A clean, healthy, and well-maintained space is a significant contribution to the safety of your workouts.

Equipment You'll Need

It can seem overwhelming when you start balancing exercises because you do not know where to begin. A great starting point is gathering the right equipment. When you have the necessary gear, machinery, and technology, your psyche pushes you to get over the hump of the first session. The equipment will enhance the effectiveness of the exercises and keep you safe. Just as a plumber needs his tools to fix a burst pipe, you must have the right equipment to keep your health in tip-top condition. Although balance exercises are versatile enough to be performed with minimal equipment, having some assistance from fitness technology will propel you forward even further. Even if the exercises are stripped down to their bare bones, there is still a need for some basic equipment to get going.

The first purchase you are likely to make is clothing. You need flexible and breathable material that is easy to move in and does not have loose hanging parts that can get snagged in the gym equipment. You will need comfortable sneakers that allow you to move your feet freely and are soft on your feet. For shoes, it is better to opt for high-quality sports brands that will last longer with foam technology that molds to your foot shape and comfortably supports your joints. Cheaper brands can sometimes have lower-quality materials that will adversely impact you in the long run.

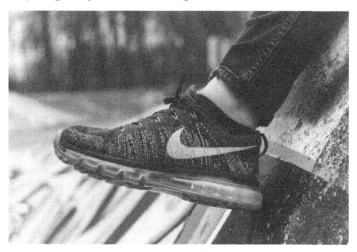

4. *You will need comfortable sneakers that allow you to move your feet freely and are soft on your feet. Source: https://www.pexels.com/photo/close-up-photography-of-red-and-black-nike-running-shoe-786003/*

Balancing exercises can be tricky at times. One of the key benefits of doing these activities is to become strong on your feet and fight the fear of falling. Therefore, you do not want to reinforce that fear in the gym. Having supports nearby, like mounted railings or free-standing rails to lean on, could be helpful, especially for a beginner. Mounts and supports can help you build confidence when you are starting and are useful in many simple exercises. Depending on your available space, your supports can be movable or fixed. Remember, you must begin slowly, so using bolters and mounts is the perfect place to start. As you progress, you will rely less on the support, but having them near could comfort you to continue fearlessly.

Resistance bands are a low-cost piece of equipment that can greatly enlarge the scope of your exercises. Unlike many other weights, resistance bands are generally safe for beginners and can be used for mild, moderate, and intense workouts. Resistance bands also have varying tension levels, so you can find what works best and which bands suit various workout regimens. These are some of the first pieces of equipment you should embrace because they are versatile and cheap. One exercise can be radically shifted simply by adding or changing the resistance bands. Resistance bands target many parts of the body and seamlessly mesh with a multitude of balance-focused workouts.

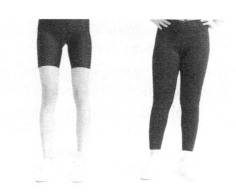

5. *Resistance bands are a low-cost piece of equipment that can greatly enlarge the scope of your exercises. Source: https://www.pexels.com/photo/people-workout-using-resistance-bands-6516206/*

Wide platforms are helpful when your balance is not the greatest. Some exercises require using a step. If the step platform is big, you have more wiggle room for mistakes and miscalculations as a beginner. Moreover, there is increased stability, so you have more freedom of movement. Some steps are adjustable so that they can be set to your body size and fitness level. Platforms and steps are perfect for getting your knees involved in an exercise, so your balance exercise can incorporate work on the joints, providing relief from stiffness. For an elderly person, you should get a step with cushioning and rounded corners. A step with a quality grip will prevent slips that could cause serious injury. For optimal results, your surface should be solid, absorb shock, be wide, and textured.

Pneumatic equipment is gym machinery using air for resistance. A variety of pneumatic devices are available on the market to cater to all fitness levels. These devices allow a wide range of assisted motion. Their designs are comfortable and adaptable for numerous workouts. Pneumatic machinery is expensive, so it is not the best option if you have budgetary restrictions. Buying pneumatic exercise machines is only advisable if you are committed due to the significant investment that goes into buying one of these advanced machines. Furthermore, you will need professional assistance to get the most out of pneumatic devices because guidance is needed to effectively and safely use complex equipment. Setting up the device could also be a hurdle, but once it is up and running, the possibilities for growth are endless.

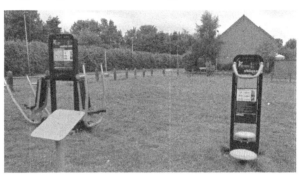

6. *Pneumatic equipment is gym machinery using air for resistance. Source: Outdoor gym equipment by Mat Fascione, CC BY-SA 2.0 <https://creativecommons.org/licenses/by-sa/2.0>, via Wikimedia Commons: https://commons.wikimedia.org/wiki/File:Outdoor_gym_equipme nt_-_geograph.org.uk_-_5490513.jpg*

Computerized training equipment like fitness watches lets you track your vital signs, ensuring you are safe. Some watches measure everything from your heart rate and oxygen level in your blood to the number of steps you walk and the calories you've burnt. The watches have timers and various modes applicable to your workouts. The information that computerized training equipment records can be relayed to your doctor so you can be advised about the best practices and safety considerations you must make during exercise. Furthermore, the data can be used to shape your diet and other exercise routines outside of the balance exercises you do. An electronic fitness watch is a nifty health tool that can be a matrix from which you plan your health activities.

Mats, cushion supports, and foam rollers allow you to adapt to various positions. There are many awkward movements in balance exercises. You may require some added comfort, especially in positions you are not used to. Having soft equipment available provides the assistance needed for exercises you may be unable to complete without their additional support. Your versatility in the gym can be increased with strategically placed mats, cushions, and foam rollers.

Choosing the Right Exercise Space

Just as the kitchen is for cooking and your bedroom is for sleeping, having a dedicated space for working out can be a motivating force when you enter the room. You have the freedom to create a room specifically catered to your needs and crafted to get the most out of you for every session. Since this text focuses on balance, your gym should be geared toward maximizing the effectiveness of your balance exercises.

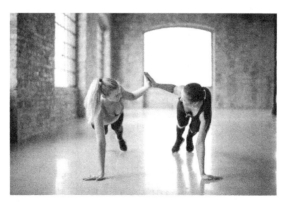

7. *When you create an exercise space, you should ensure that you can get in and out of it easily. Source: https://www.pexels.com/photo/young-slender-female-athletes-giving-high-five-to-each-other-while-training-together-in-sports-club-3768722/*

Mobility can be an issue, especially in unfamiliar places. Therefore, when you create an exercise space, you should ensure that you can get in and out of it easily. For example, if you have trouble climbing stairs, you cannot have a gym room at the top of a building. You must be able to travel easily to and from your exercise space. Some people walk assisted using walkers or vanes, so you must factor in this variable. Having clear access to your space and navigating it freely will add to how comfortable you are in your gym.

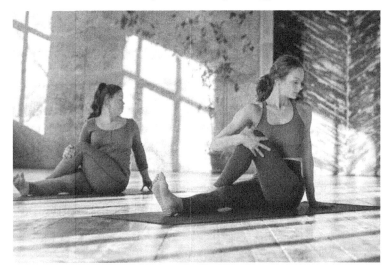

8. *Comfort is key when putting together your exercise space. Source: https://www.pexels.com/photo/photo-of-women-stretching-together-4056723/*

Comfort is key when putting together your exercise space. From the temperature to the decor, your comfort inside the room should be catered to at every level. You do not need an excuse to stay away, so create a functional gym space you want to spend hours within. If you need to rest between sets or do exercises sitting down, have comfortable chairs readily available. If you require assistance walking, railings could do wonders for the space. You have unique needs, so think about what will create the most positive experience. Your comfort comes first because you do not want to sustain injuries due to being put in an unfavorable environment.

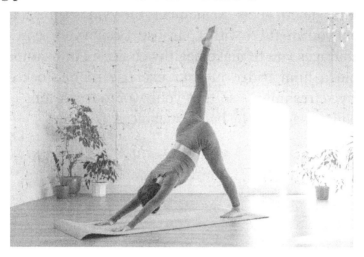

9. *Ideally, you want an open and uncluttered space with a lot of light where you can move freely. Source:*
https://www.pexels.com/photo/a-woman-doing-stretching-exercise-6648788/

Ideally, you want an open and uncluttered space with a lot of light where you can move freely. Obstructions in the gym do not only inhibit your progress, but they can also be safety hazards. All your equipment should be spaced out well to allow walking and moving freely. In case you fall, there should not be objects in the way where you can severely hurt yourself. A spacious gym is optimal for balance exercises, so make sure that whichever room you set up for exercising has enough open space to use your body freely and embrace the exaggerated movements balance exercises sometimes require.

Your exercise space should be clean and healthy. A moldy, dusty room will only make you ill, which directly opposes your mission to increase your well-being in your later years. Sanitizers and towels are a brilliant addition to a gym. Keeping your space clean makes the gym hygienic and inviting. You should always want to be inside the space you have set up for exercising, and you want the space to mesh with your health goals. Remember, the gym is a place to have fun, but you are there with a purpose. Design your gym so that it encourages you to make healthy choices. For example, you can put a mini fridge in your exercise room stocked with healthy refreshments so that your workout sessions are not immediately spoiled by bad diet choices.

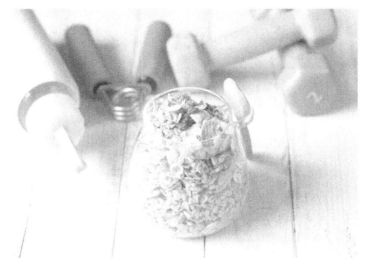

10. Your focus is exercising for balance, but a holistic workout approach will have the best results. Source: https://unsplash.com/photos/clear-glass-jar-with-brown-powder-YJzCsH3QjS4

Add a variety of equipment to your exercise room. Your focus is exercising for balance, but a holistic workout approach will have the best results. Set up cardio and strength stations combined with the foam rollers, steps, and resistance bands for balancing. Switching up your routine will keep your workouts interesting. Do not be one-dimensional in the room, but rather embrace a variety that motivates you to get into the numerous activities that alleviate age-related ailments. The more options you have, the more likely you will remain consistent because you will not get bored with the repetition.

Your physical well-being is not the only sphere of yourself that your gym should be catering to. Staying consistent with exercise requires mental devotion. If you go into any fighting gym, famous legends and inspirational sayings will be plastered all over the walls. Coaches understand that fighters must be in the correct state of mind to train and perform optimally. Therefore, the psychology of the room should be taken into account. Calming colors and a mirror are two style choices that can be motivating. A mirror helps you maintain good form and allows you to see the work you put in. The colors in the room can create the exact feeling you resonate with the most.

Chapter 3: Warm-Up and Stretching

Warming up your body before balance exercises is imperative as it primes the body and prepares it to perform exercises effectively. A warm-up before exercise increases the heart rate and gets the blood flowing to every muscle, prepping them for intense activity. These warm-ups improve joint mobility, activate specific muscle groups, and decrease muscle stiffness. The effects of warm-ups prevent injuries. On the other hand, stretching reduces muscle tension, increases the body's flexibility, and enables a greater range of motion. Together, warm-ups and stretching exercises protect you from injuries, make muscles more responsive, significantly improve muscle control, and maintain stability.

Importance of Warm-Up

Whether it's a weight-lifting workout or simple balance exercises, regardless of the exercise, it's always necessary to warm up the body and prepare it before starting the physical activity. Here's why warm-ups are essential before every exercise, especially balance exercises:

Increased Blood Flow

Warm-up exercises gradually elevate your heart rate and increase blood circulation, essential for seniors, ensuring your muscles receive adequate oxygen and nutrients. Improved blood flow prepares your body for the increased demands of balance exercises and reduces the risk of cardiovascular stress during the workout. Cold muscles receive less oxygen and fewer nutrients, leading to inefficient blood flow. It can result in early muscle fatigue during balance exercises, limiting the duration and quality of the workout. Seniors need help to sustain exercises for extended periods, diminishing the potential benefits of their efforts.

Enhanced Joint Lubrication

Joint mobility can decrease with age, potentially leading to stiffness and discomfort. Warm-up activities involve gentle, controlled movements that help lubricate your joints by stimulating the production of synovial fluid. This lubrication eases joint movement, making maintaining proper posture and alignment easier during balance exercises.

Doing warm-up activities stimulates the production of synovial fluid in the joints naturally. The fluid acts as a lubricant, facilitating pain-free movement and cushioning the joints to protect them from injuries. Seniors who skip warm-ups could experience less effective joint lubrication, leading to discomfort, stiffness, and potentially more wear and tear on their joints.

Prevention of Injuries

One of the primary benefits of a warm-up is injury prevention. Seniors are more prone to muscle strains, joint injuries, and falls during exercise due to decreased flexibility and muscle elasticity. A proper warm-up readies your muscles and connective tissues for physical activity, reducing the risk of strains, tears, or sprains during balance exercises.

When you skip warm-up exercises, the muscles, tendons, and ligaments aren't adequately prepared for the demands of balance exercises. Cold and stiff tissues are more vulnerable to injuries like muscle strains, joint sprains, or ligament tears. These injuries can be painful and debilitating and require extended recovery periods, potentially discouraging you from continuing the exercise routine.

Improved Neuromuscular Coordination

Warm-ups are crucial in enhancing neuromuscular coordination, the connection between your muscles and nervous system. Maintaining solid connections between muscles and nerves becomes crucial for maintaining balance and stability as you age.

Warm-up exercises activate these connections, improving your body's ability to respond effectively to balance challenges. An inadequate warm-up can result in reduced coordination, making it more challenging for seniors to respond effectively to balance challenges. It increases the risk of falls and diminishes the overall quality of their workouts.

Mental Readiness

Warm-ups shift your focus to the task, mentally preparing you for exercise. This mental readiness is particularly valuable for seniors, as it promotes concentration and mindfulness during balance exercises. Being mentally engaged reduces the likelihood of accidents or missteps, enhancing overall safety. Warm-ups serve as a transition from a passive state to an active one.

They mentally prepare individuals for exercise, helping them shift their focus and adopt a mental attitude conducive to physical activity. Seniors who skip warm-ups find it harder to concentrate and maintain mindfulness during balance exercises, reducing their ability to perform safely and effectively.

Reduction in Muscle Stiffness

Aging can increase muscle stiffness, making it challenging to move fluidly and maintain balance. Warm-up routines alleviate muscle stiffness by gradually increasing muscle temperature. This helps you perform balance exercises with greater fluidity, control, and range of motion.

Avoiding Warm-Ups

Besides the problems mentioned above from avoiding warm-ups, here are other issues that occur when you avoid a good warm-up before exercise.

Reduced Flexibility

Naturally, aging leads to a decrease in joint flexibility and mobility. Cold muscles and joints are less supple, making it challenging to perform balance exercises with a full range of motion. This restricted mobility compromises exercise form and decreases the workout's effectiveness.

Increased Recovery Time

Injuries or discomfort stemming from inadequate warm-up can lead to longer recovery periods. Extended recovery disrupts the consistency of an exercise routine, potentially causing frustration or demotivation. An extended recovery period can be particularly discouraging and can lead to abandoning regular exercise altogether.

Diminished Workout Benefits

Warm-ups prepare the body for the physical demands of exercise. With proper preparation, seniors fully reap the benefits of their balance exercises. An insufficient warm-up limits the range of motion, stability, and muscle engagement during the workout. Consequently, the effectiveness of the exercise is compromised, and progress becomes slower or less noticeable.

Loss of Exercise Enjoyment

Unpleasant or uncomfortable exercise experiences due to the absence of warm-ups can deter anyone from engaging in regular physical activity. It quickly leads to reluctance or resistance toward maintaining an active lifestyle.

Warm-up exercises are a critical step for anyone following a fitness routine. These warm-up routines and exercises not only aid in improving physical fitness but also keep metabolic processes at an optimum rate. Each benefit of warm-up exercises collectively limits the risk of injuries and improves balance. Seniors who incorporate warm-ups into their exercise regimen are likelier to enjoy safer, more effective, and more enjoyable balance workouts, reaping the numerous benefits of enhanced mobility and stability.

Warm-Ups to Follow

Ankle Circles

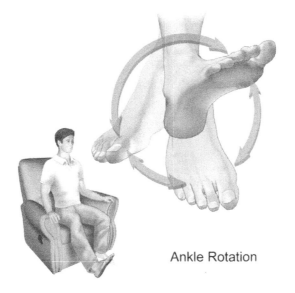

Ankle Rotation

11. This warms up the ankle joints and improves ankle mobility, vital for balance. Source: BruceBlaus, CC BY-SA 4.0 <https://creativecommons.org/licenses/by-sa/4.0>, via Wikimedia Commons: https://commons.wikimedia.org/wiki/File:Exercise_Ankle_Rotation.png

1. Sit on a chair or stand with your feet flat on the floor.

2. Lift one foot slightly off the ground.

3. Rotate your ankle in a circular motion, clockwise for 15 seconds and counterclockwise for 15 seconds.

4. Repeat with the other ankle.

This warms up the ankle joints and improves ankle mobility, vital for balance.

March in Place

1. Stand with your feet hip-width apart.

2. Lift your knees alternately, as if marching, while gently swinging your arms.

3. Continue for 30 seconds to 1 minute.

This increases heart rate and gets the blood flowing to the lower body.

Arm Circles

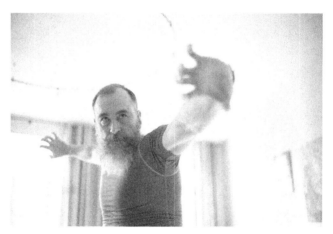

12. *This exercise activates the shoulder joints and improves upper body mobility. Source: https://www.pexels.com/photo/bearded-man-stretching-arms-6975767/*

1. Stand with your feet shoulder-width apart.

2. Extend your arms straight out to the sides.

3. Make small circles with your arms, clockwise for 15 seconds and then counterclockwise for 15 seconds.

4. Gradually increase the size of the circles.

This exercise activates the shoulder joints and improves upper body mobility.

Leg Swings

1. Stand beside a sturdy support, like a chair or wall, for balance.

2. Swing one leg forward and backward, gently increasing the range of motion.

3. Perform 10-15 swings with each leg.

The hip and leg muscles get activated with these leg swings.

Shoulder Rolls

1. Stand with your feet hip-width apart.

2. Roll your shoulders forward in a circular motion for 15 seconds.

3. Then, roll them backward for 15 seconds.

The exercise relaxes the shoulder muscles and improves joint mobility.

Torso Twists

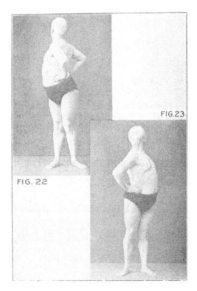

13. The core muscles are activated in this exercise, improving spinal mobility and core strength. Source: https://commons.wikimedia.org/wiki/File:Tensing_Exercises_Fig 22.jpg

1. Stand with your feet hip-width apart and arms extended straight before you.

2. Rotate your torso to one side and then the other, using your hips as a pivot point.

3. Perform 10-15 twists on each side.

The core muscles are activated in this exercise, improving spinal mobility and core strength.

High Knees

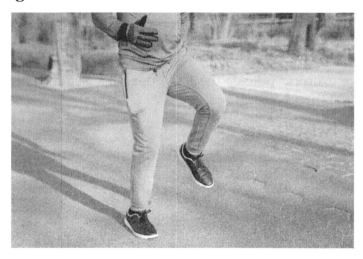

14. *It has a similar effect to leg swings, activating the leg muscles and joints of the leg, especially the knee. Source: https://www.pexels.com/photo/crop-unrecognizable-sportsman-jumping-on-one-leg-7869578/*

1. Stand with your feet hip-width apart.

2. Lift one knee as high as comfortable, then switch to the other knee in a marching motion.

3. Continue for 30 seconds to 1 minute.

It has a similar effect to leg swings, activating the leg muscles and joints of the leg, especially the knee.

Heel Raises

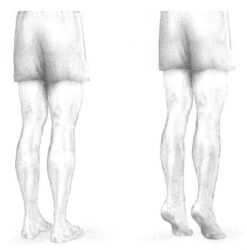

Two Leg Heel Raise

15. This is one of the best warm-up exercises for calf muscles. Source: BruceBlaus, CC BY-SA 4.0 <https://creativecommons.org/licenses/by-sa/4.0>, via Wikimedia Commons: https://commons.wikimedia.org/wiki/File:Exercise_Heel_Raise_Two_Legs.png

1. Keep the feet broad apart while standing.

2. Lift up the heels while keeping the toes on the ground.

3. After a total elevation, slowly lower the heels.

4. Perform the heel raises for at least 30 seconds to a minute.

This is one of the best warm-up exercises for calf muscles and can increase ankle stability, making it easier to maintain balance.

Wrist Circles

1. Sit or stand with your arms extended in front of you.

2. Make circular motions with your wrists, clockwise for 15 seconds and then counterclockwise for 15 seconds.

This exercise warms up the wrist muscles and joints, improving wrist mobility while performing exercises.

Deep Breathing

1. Stand or sit in a comfortable position.

2. Take slow, deep breaths, inhaling through your nose and exhaling through your mouth.

3. Continue for 1-2 minutes.

Just as you activate the body physically, this deep breathing exercise keeps the body relaxed and clears the mind.

The Difference between Stretching and Warm-Ups

Think of warm-ups as the initial phase of your pre-exercise routine. Warm-up exercises prepare the body for physical activity, including the muscles, joints, and related organs. Most warm-ups are performed before an exercise session, lasting from ten to fifteen minutes. The main objectives of a warm-up routine are to increase the heart rate for optimum blood flow, especially to the targeted muscles, elevate the body temperature, and prime the body for a more physically intense activity.

Most warm-up exercises include aerobic exercises, jogging, cycling, brisk walking, yoga, low-intensity practices, and specific exercises to target muscle groups, like the balance exercises described earlier in the chapter. Warm-up exercises are primarily organized in an order, from low-intensity exercises to moderate ones. This practice slowly warms the body, gradually elevating the heart rate and breathing without causing fatigue. Furthermore, warm-ups are critical in enhancing joint mobility and activating the muscles for physically demanding exercises.

On the contrary, stretching is a distinct component of a pre- and post-exercise routine with the primary objective of extending the range of motion in several muscle groups and increasing flexibility. Stretches can be performed as a part of warm-ups or as a separate activity before or after the exercise. While there are several stretching techniques, the three basic ones include static stretching, dynamic stretching, and proprioceptive neuromuscular facilitation (PNF) stretching.

Stretching exercises are low-intensity and should not cause pain or discomfort. The focus of stretching is on gradually increasing muscle length and improving joint flexibility. Stretching helps alleviate muscle tension and reduces the risk of musculoskeletal injuries, like strains or muscle imbalances. It is highly specific, targeting particular muscles or muscle groups, and can be customized based on individual flexibility and mobility needs.

While warm-ups and stretching are essential components of a pre-exercise routine, they serve distinct purposes. Warm-ups prepare the entire body for physical activity by increasing circulation, heart rate, and mental readiness and reducing the risk of injury. Stretching focuses on improving muscle flexibility and joint range of motion in specific areas. It is done as part of the warm-up or independently to enhance overall mobility and reduce the risk of muscle-related injuries.

Stretching Exercises for Seniors

Neck Stretch

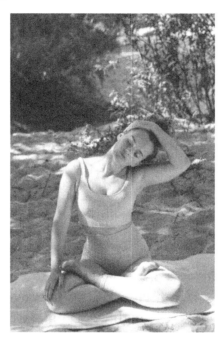

16. This exercise helps relieve tension in the neck and improves neck flexibility. Source: https://www.pexels.com/photo/a-woman-in-activewear-stretching-her-neck-8534776/

1. Have a straight back while you sit or stand.

2. Bring your ear near your shoulder as you slowly tilt your head to one side.

3. The other side of your neck ought to feel slightly stretched.

4. Maintain this posture for 15 to 30 seconds.

5. Perform the same stretch on the opposing side.

This exercise helps relieve tension in the neck and improves neck flexibility.

Shoulder Stretch

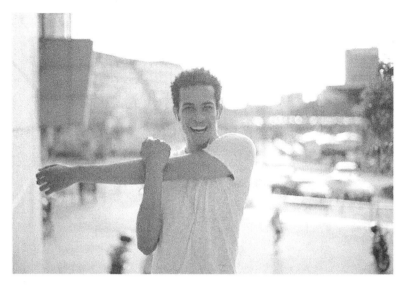

17. These shoulder stretches relax the shoulder muscles and improve shoulder mobility. Source: https://www.pexels.com/photo/happy-young-ethnic-sportsman-stretching-arms-while-warming-up-before-training-on-street-in-city-3799256/

1. Reach one arm across your chest.

2. Use your opposite hand to pull your arm closer to your chest gently.

3. You should feel a stretch in the back of your shoulder.

4. Hold for 15-30 seconds.

5. Repeat the stretch with the other arm.

These shoulder stretches relax the shoulder muscles and improve shoulder mobility.

Triceps Stretch

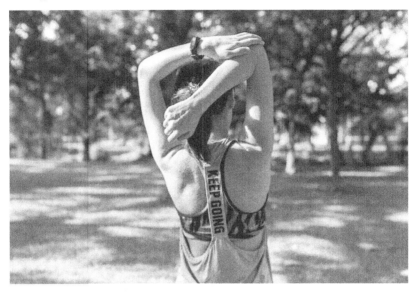

18. The triceps stretch improves triceps flexibility, making the arms coordinate better. Source: https://www.pexels.com/photo/unrecognizable-female-athlete-stretching-muscles-of-arms-and-back-4426321/ Raise one arm over your head, bend the elbow, and extend your hand down your spine.

1. Use your opposite hand to push your bent elbow gently.

2. You should feel a stretch along the back of your upper arm (triceps).

3. Hold for 30 seconds.

4. Repeat the stretch with the other arm.

The triceps stretch improves triceps flexibility, making the arms coordinate better.

Chest Opener

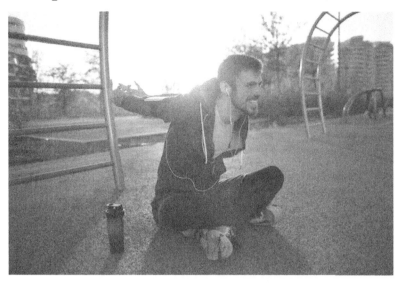

*19. This stretch is an excellent way to counteract a hunched back.
Source: https://www.pexels.com/photo/cheerful-athletic-man-
stretching-arms-on-sports-ground-3771094/*

1. Keeping the feet shoulder-wide apart, clasp your hands behind your back.

2. Slightly bend your elbows and lift your arms, opening your chest.

3. You should feel a stretch across your chest and shoulders.

4. Hold for half a minute.

This stretch is an excellent way to counteract a hunched back. It becomes easier for your body to coordinate better and improve balance by doing these stretches.

Back Stretch

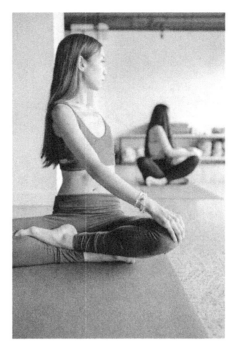

20. The spinal flexibility improves greatly with this back stretch exercise. Source: https://www.pexels.com/photo/woman-in-gray-crop-top-and-leggings-on-a-yoga-mat-8436709/

1. Sit on a chair with your feet flat on the floor.

2. Slowly twist your torso to one side while keeping your hips facing forward.

3. You should feel a gentle stretch in your back and spine.

4. Hold for 15 to 30 seconds.

5. Repeat the stretch on the other side.

The spinal flexibility improves greatly with this back stretch exercise.

Quadriceps Stretch

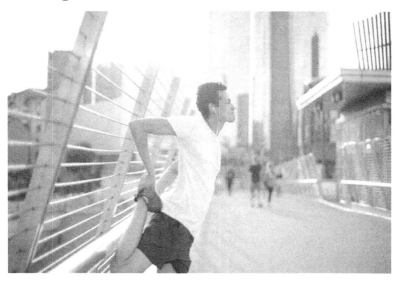

21. This stretch targets the front thigh muscles, improving the leg muscles' strength and priming them to perform effectively. Source: https://www.pexels.com/photo/focused-millennial-ethnic-athlete-in-earphones-listening-to-music-and-stretching-body-before-running-on-street-3799375/

1. While standing, hold onto a stable surface, like a chair, to maintain balance.

2. Bend one knee and bring your heel toward your buttocks.

3. Use your hand to hold your ankle or foot.

4. You should feel a stretch in the front of your thigh (quadriceps).

5. Stay in the position for 15-30 seconds.

6. Repeat the stretch with the other leg.

This stretch targets the front thigh muscles, improving the leg muscles' strength and priming them to perform effectively.

Hamstring Stretch

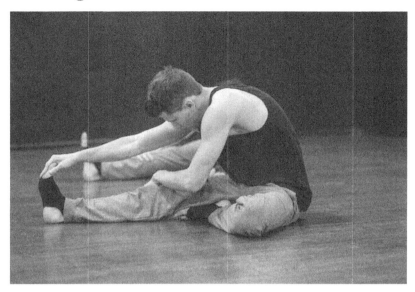

22. This stretch exercise improves the hamstring's flexibility. Source: https://www.pexels.com/photo/a-man-doing-a-hamstring-stretch-6926025/

1. Sit on the edge of a chair with one leg extended straight and the other foot flat on the floor.

2. Lean forward from your hips while keeping your back straight.

3. You should feel a stretch in the back of your thigh (hamstring).

4. Hold for 15-30 seconds.

5. Repeat the stretch with the other leg.

This stretch exercise improves the hamstring's flexibility, supporting the knee during movement.

Calf Stretch

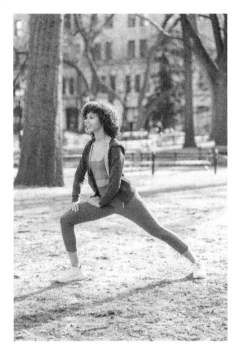

23. This stretch targets the calf muscles. Source: https://www.pexels.com/photo/fit-black-woman-stretching-legs-in-park-in-daylight-7242895/

1. Stand facing a wall with your hands on the wall at shoulder height.

2. Step one foot back and press your heel into the floor.

3. Keep your back leg straight and your front knee slightly bent.

4. Lean your upper body forward.

5. You should feel a stretch in the calf muscle.

6. Hold for 15-30 seconds.

7. Switch to the other leg.

This stretch targets the calf muscles.

Ankle Circles

1. Sit on a chair with your feet flat on the floor.

2. Lift one foot and gently rotate your ankle in a clockwise motion.

3. After 15-30 seconds, switch to counterclockwise rotation.

4. Repeat the same ankle circles with the other foot.

This exercise helps improve ankle flexibility and mobility.

Wrist Flexor Stretch

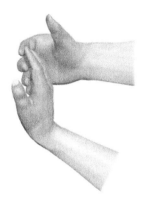

Wrist Flexor Stretch

24. This stretch targets the wrist and forearm muscles. Source: BruceBlaus, CC BY-SA 4.0 <https://creativecommons.org/licenses/by-sa/4.0>, via Wikimedia Commons: https://commons.wikimedia.org/wiki/File:Exercise_Wrist_Flexor_Stretch.png

1. Extend one arm in front of you at shoulder height.

2. Point your fingers upward and gently pull them back with your opposite hand.

3. You should feel a stretch in the front of your forearm.

4. Hold for 15-30 seconds.

5. Repeat the stretch with the other hand.

This stretch targets the wrist and forearm muscles.

Hip Flexor Stretch

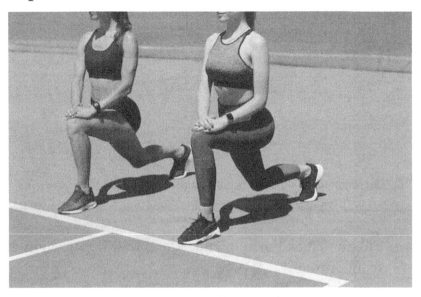

25. This exercise helps improve hip flexor flexibility. Source: https://www.pexels.com/photo/two-women-doing-stretching-4348626/

1. Stand or kneel with one foot forward and the other foot extended behind you.

2. Keep your back straight and engage your core.

3. Shift your weight forward slightly, feeling a stretch in the front of your hip on the extended leg.

4. Hold for 15-30 seconds.

5. Repeat the stretch with the other leg.

This exercise helps improve hip flexor flexibility.

Inner Thigh Stretch

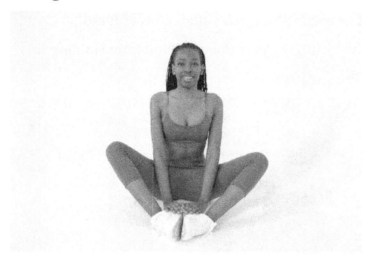

26. The inner thigh muscles become more flexible with this stretch. Source: https://www.pexels.com/photo/fit-black-woman-sitting-in-baddha-konasana-pose-6311694/

1. Take a seat on the floor and extend your legs straight in front of you.

2. Bring the soles of your feet together and bend your knees.

3. Feel for a stretch in your inner thighs as you gently press your knees toward the floor.

4. Hold this position for 15 to 30 seconds.

5. You can gently push your knees for a deeper stretch with your hands.

The inner thigh muscles become more flexible with this stretch.

Outer Thigh Stretch

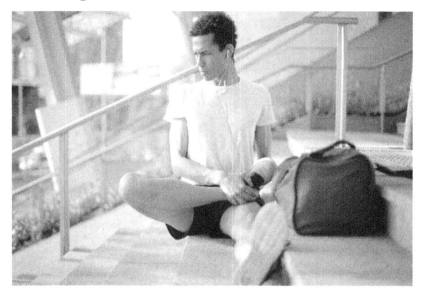

*27. The hip and outer thigh muscles are worked during this exercise.
Source: https://www.pexels.com/photo/young-ethnic-athlete-in-earbuds-stretching-body-while-sitting-on-stairs-at-entrance-of-contemporary-building-3799277/*

1. Place your feet flat on the ground while sitting in a chair.

2. Place one ankle over the knee of the other.

3. Feel for a stretch in the outer thigh and hip as you gently press down on the elevated knee.

4. Hold this position for 15 to 30 seconds.

5. Repeat the exercise with the other leg.

The hip and outer thigh muscles are worked during this exercise.

Calf and Achilles Stretch (Wall Stretch)

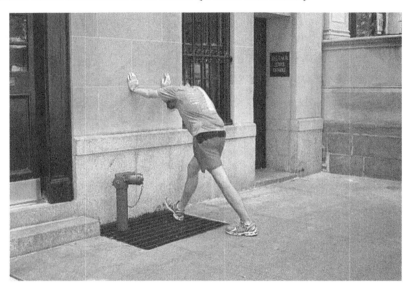

28. This stretch improves calf and Achilles tendon flexibility. Source: Timothy Krause, CC BY 2.0 <https://creativecommons.org/licenses/by/2.0>, via Wikimedia Commons: https://commons.wikimedia.org/wiki/File:Stretching_(755923407 2).jpg

1. Stand facing a wall and place your hands against it.

2. Step one foot back and press your heel into the floor.

3. Keep your back leg straight and your front knee slightly bent.

4. Lean your upper body forward, feeling a stretch in your calf and Achilles tendon.

5. Hold for 15-30 seconds.

6. Switch to the other leg.

This stretch improves calf and Achilles tendon flexibility.

Seated Toe Touch

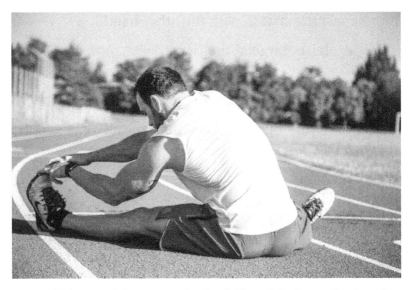

29. This stretch improves the flexibility of the lower back and hamstrings. Source: Source: https://unsplash.com/photos/man-in-white-sleeveless-top-WX7FSaiYxK8

1. Take a seat on the floor and extend your legs straight in front of you.

2. Reach forward slowly, attempting to touch your shins or toes.

3. Avoid hunching your back or rounding your spine.

4. Hold the position for 15 to 30 seconds.

This stretch improves the flexibility of the lower back and hamstrings.

Wrist Extensor Stretch

1. Extend one arm in front of you at shoulder height.

2. Point your fingers downward and gently pull them back with your opposite hand.

3. You should feel a stretch in the back of your forearm.

4. Hold for 15-30 seconds.

5. Repeat the stretch with the other hand.

This exercise targets the wrist and forearm extensor muscles.

Standing Quadriceps Stretch

1. Stand with one hand against a wall or a chair for balance.

2. Bend your knee and bring your heel toward your buttocks.

3. Use your hand to hold your ankle or foot.

4. You should feel a stretch in the front of your thigh (quadriceps).

5. Hold for 15-30 seconds.

6. Repeat the stretch with the other leg.

This exercise targets the quadriceps muscles.

Side Stretch

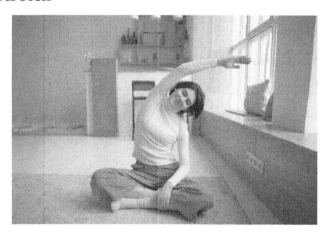

30. This stretch improves lateral flexibility. Source: https://www.pexels.com/photo/smiling-woman-practicing-yoga-with-closed-eyes-at-home-4051507/

1. Stand with your feet shoulder-width apart.

2. Raise one arm overhead and gently lean to the opposite side.

3. Keep your feet planted firmly on the ground.

4. You should feel a stretch along the side of your torso.

5. Hold for 15-30 seconds on each side.

This stretch improves lateral flexibility.

Child's Pose (for Flexibility and Relaxation)

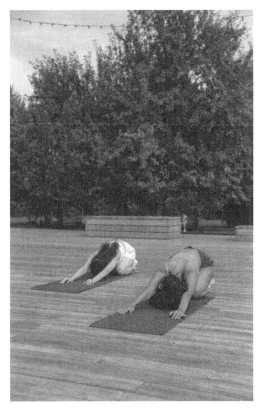

31.   This exercise promotes relaxation, stretches the back, and improves flexibility in the spine. Source: https://www.pexels.com/photo/faceless-women-practicing-extended-childs-pose-in-nature-5384557/

1. Start in a kneeling position with your big toes touching.

2. Sit back onto your heels and stretch your arms forward.

3. Bend forward, rest your forehead on the ground, and relax.

4. Hold for 15-30 seconds.

This exercise promotes relaxation, stretches the back, and improves flexibility in the spine.

These stretching exercises for seniors can be easily incorporated into the daily routine to enhance flexibility, reduce muscle tension, and promote overall mobility. It's essential to perform each stretch slowly and gently without pushing beyond a comfortable range of motion. If seniors have existing medical conditions or concerns, they should consult a healthcare professional or fitness expert before starting a new stretching regimen.

Chapter 4: Balance Building Exercises

Having gained an in-depth understanding of the science of balance, what you need to get started, and warming up and stretching properly, you are now ready to learn some basic exercises. These workouts are specifically for gaining strength, stability, and flexibility. The exercises are simple to understand and consider your limitations. Creating a routine that includes even a few of these exercises will have enough impact to shift your quality of life significantly. The instructions are easy to understand with visual representations so you can see the perfect form and gauge what your body will allow.

The CDCP (the Centers for Disease Control and Prevention) recommends that people over 65 should exercise at least 150 minutes a week. The time can be split in various ways, but for simplicity, they can be calculated at 30 minutes a day from Monday to Friday. The techniques listed below should be kept fresh and engaging because they can create a dynamic gym regime. Many people give up pursuing their health goals because the processes are tedious and repetitious.

You will find what works for you because many workout variations are outlined for a wide range of capabilities.

Your entire body will be engaged with gentle work targeting all your muscle groups. You have a selection of options waiting for you to explore, from standing exercises and gentle stretches to chair workouts and active motion. Listen to your body, be careful, follow medical advice, and find what works best for you. These exercises can supplement your current schedule, or they can be used to create an entirely new routine. A little goes a long way, so do not try to get everything done at once. Break down muscle groups into sections, give yourself time to rest to avoid injury, and stick to your balance-reinforcing exercise journey.

Standing Exercises

Marching on the Spot

Balance has a lot to do with motion. Your vestibular system works by receiving input based on how you navigate space. Therefore, an exercise that includes motion is helpful to keep your balance in tip-top shape. You do not have to get overcomplicated at first. Marching on the spot is a great exercise that combines cardio, balance, and the movement of your joints. Moreover, the motion stimulates the mechanism of your inner ear, so you get used to moving around. The little things you do can make significant changes. Spending a few minutes a day getting your knees up to march will make a world of difference in your overall health and wellness. Put on some music and have fun with marching as a wake-up booster in the mornings.

- Be careful, but see how high you can lift your legs and how far you can swing your arms when doing this workout.

- You can change your pace to match your level of comfort.

- Start marching for two minutes a day, then gradually increase to five minutes.

- Over time, you can push it to as long as ten to fifteen minutes.

Toe Lifts

Toe lifts are perfect for engaging your legs to improve balance.

- For this exercise, you will need a chair, table, or counter just above waist height.

- Alternatively, use a wall for support.

- Stretch your arms out in front of you and grab hold of the table or chair.

- Stand with your legs moderately apart, squared with your hips, and facing the chair.

- Slowly ascend to your tippy toes, then relax and descend until flat-footed again.

- Repeat this exercise about ten times in each repetition.

- You will feel your calves and thighs tighten when you do this exercise.

Rocking the Boat

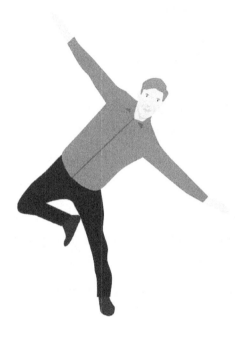

32. Rocking the boat is a simple exercise that uses motion to increase strength, balance, and fitness. However, it is a lot less strenuous than marching on the spot. Source: https://pixabay.com/illustrations/arms-fly-balancing-idea-like-2938764/

- Start by standing with your legs at about hip-width apart.

- Spread your toes to the ground and onto the floor with stability.

- Now, shift your weight slowly onto your right leg while raising your left leg.

- Alternate between each leg and make sure to move slowly and deliberately, feeling every muscle and how the bones in your feet adjust to movement.

- Hold your balance on each leg for ten to twenty seconds.

Single Leg Stands

Back Leg Raises

This exercise requires a chair or another stabilizing support, like a rail or walker. The extra support will secure you so that you can embrace being on one leg without the fear of falling. Exercises that alternate between each leg help you isolate the individual muscles in your lower body so you can deeply feel which areas get engaged when working out. This simple and safe exercise is amazing to get the blood flowing from your hips to your toes.

- Stretch your hands out in front of you and grab hold of the chair.

- Stand in a wide stance with your feet facing straight forward and in line with your hips.

- Take a few breaths and get comfortable in the position.

- Keeping your leg straight, raise your right foot toward your back, facing your heel up to the ceiling.

- See how far you can move your leg and stop when you can't lift it any higher.

- Do ten repetitions on each leg, alternating between every rep.

- This exercise targets your lower back, hamstrings, and glutes (the groups of muscles in your buttocks).

- In addition to helping with balance, this workout can alleviate lower back pain.

Single Limb Stance

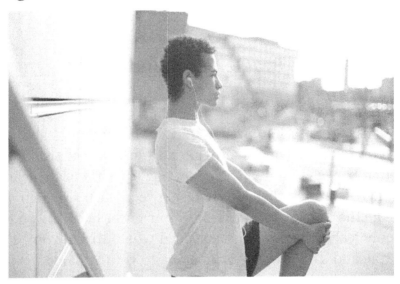

33. Balance is a full-body activity with minor adjustments to your joints and muscles to maintain an upright position. Source: https://www.pexels.com/photo/focused-millennial-ethnic-sportsman-in-earbuds-listening-to-music-and-warming-up-alone-on-street-in-downtown-3799246/

Balance is a full-body activity with minor adjustments to your joints and muscles to maintain an upright position. For these muscles to work together, you need coordination. The single-limb stance coupled with arm movement is brilliant for building much-needed coordination to create a unified body. When you understand the interconnectivity of the body, you realize that multiple muscles and tendons play a role in balance. Getting your arms and legs working together introduces you to the intricacies of how different parts of your body work together to achieve specific goals. Furthermore, using various muscle combinations increases the intensity and effectiveness of your workout. The multiple muscles and joints used in this exercise will get you working up a healthy sweat.

- Position the back of a chair or a rail next to you.

- You can swap the chair for a table or counter to support your weight.

- Slowly lift your left arm while stabilizing yourself with your right hand on the chair.

- Once your arm is in the air, lift the opposite leg, moving your knee toward your chest.

- Alternate this exercise between each leg.

Single-Foot Balance

When you do dynamic movements in daily life, you'll often stand in awkward positions, shifting your center of gravity from one foot to the other. Miscalculations based on a lack of training and familiarity with your body can cause disastrous falls. Doing single-foot balance workouts in a safe space can be life-changing because it strengthens both sides of your body individually. Furthermore, the slow, deliberate movements of the exercise reestablish a mind and body bond that can be lost with age as people move around less.

- For this exercise, place a chair next to you for balance.

- Stand with your feet facing straight forward and your back as straight as possible.

- Your posture allows you to involve your core in balancing and not to rely predominantly on your limbs.

- Slowly lift your leg, bending your knee toward your chest.

- Hold the position for about thirty seconds, then lower your leg slowly.

- Repeat three times for each leg.

- If you feel comfortable without using the chair for support, try doing this exercise without it. However, keeping the chair nearby is advisable in case you lose balance.

Heel-to-Toe Walks

Heel-to-Toe Walking

Walking is a gentle exercise that can be easily adapted for different health aims. Changing how you walk for exercise will help you calibrate your body better by connecting how your muscles react in relatively mundane activities. The gentle motions allow you to feel the little spaces between the bones of your feet and how the complex network is fine-tuned for balance. Staying on your feet is not only about big movements and large adjustments but is also about the tiny shifts made with your feet and toes. The joints in your feet and ankles become stiff as you age. To loosen these joints without injuring yourself, practice heel-to-toe walking for a few minutes daily.

- It helps to have a straight line to follow to perform a heel-to-toe walk.

- Use masking tape on the floor to create the line, or use existing lines from tiles or paving as a guide.

- Pay attention to what your feet are doing as you mindfully place one leg in front of the other on the line.

- The heel of the front foot should make contact with the line first. As you shift your weight forward, roll your foot slowly onto your toes as you step forward.

- Take about twenty steps walking with this technique.

- Focus on your feet and feel the stretch in the muscles, bones, and tiny joints in your feet.

Heel-to-Toe Rocking

This exercise is helpful and meditative. The relaxing motion helps create a connection between both sides of your feet, allowing them to work in unison. The gentle rocking back and forth releases tension in your ankles so that you can walk with much more comfort. The exercise also helps with standing and sitting up because your feet and ankles engage when completing these activities.

- Place a chair in front of you and hold onto it for balance.
- Spread your legs with your feet about hip-width apart.
- Put your weight on your heels, lifting your toes to the ceiling.
- Gently rock back and forth from on your heels onto your toes.
- Rock slowly so that you feel the engagement of your lower legs and feet.
- Rock back and forth between your toes and heels for twenty to thirty repetitions.
- This exercise helps relieve stiffness in your ankles by getting circulation into the region.
- Heel-to-toe rocking creates increased mobility, contributing to improving your balance.

Circling

- Your foot placement on the ground changes according to which direction you move.

- If you watch the training sessions of high-speed sports like basketball or soccer, you'll notice a percentage of training time is spent on moving explosively to prepare for the unpredictable movements of the game.

- You won't be expected to perform at athlete level, but slowly circling and walking along a snake-like curving path will rotate your ankle joints in various directions, allowing you to step more complexly, preparing for the movements you'll encounter in everyday life.

- Switch up the walk by making sharper and gentler turns to tap into numerous movements.

Side Leg Lifts

Side leg lifts work on multiple muscle groups simultaneously, so they can be a bit strenuous, especially for beginners. However, they are hugely beneficial. The exercise works on your glutes and obliques, so both your legs and core are involved.

- Position yourself next to a chair, counter, or table for balance.

- Extend your leg out to the side and lift it as high as possible, keeping your body straight, then lower your leg back to the ground.

- Repeat the exercise ten times on each leg.

- You will progressively balance with less support while doing this exercise if you practice it regularly.

- The activity helps stabilize your pelvis and reduce back pain.

- Make sure you consider your safety and listen to your body so you do not make the mistake of overexerting yourself and pushing beyond your limits into injury.

Lunges

When moving forward and feeling you are about to fall, you will typically stumble to regain your balance. Lunges mimic this stumbling motion and involve the same muscle groups that keep you upright in a tripping scenario. Lunges can get a sweat going, so be ready to work hard.

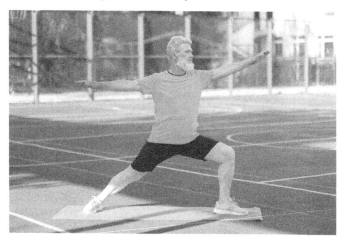

34. Lunges mimic this stumbling motion and involve the same muscle groups that keep you upright in a tripping scenario. Source: https://www.pexels.com/photo/senior-man-in-orange-shirt-and-black-pants-doing-yoga-5067957/

- Stand straight with your hands on your hips.

- Take a big step forward and bend down until your thigh is in line with the floor beneath it.

- If you cannot get your thigh parallel to the ground, just go as low as you can.

- Hold the lunge for a few seconds before returning to a standing position.

- Repeat this cycle about ten to twenty times per leg.

Seated Exercise

Sit and Stand Squat

Doing a full squat can be a bit much, especially if you have pain and inflammation in your knees. However, it is essential to work on the upper leg muscles and get the motion going in your knee joints for the sake of your balancing abilities.

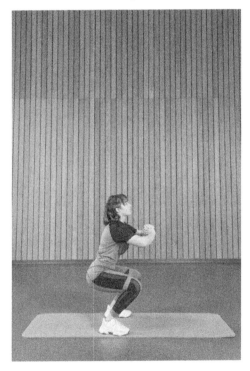

35. Doing a full squat can be a bit much, especially if you have pain and inflammation in your knees. Source: https://www.pexels.com/photo/a-woman-standing-on-a-mat-doing-the-squats-with-a-resistance-band-6339648/

- Sit down on a chair or the couch with your back straight.

- Simply stand up and sit back down.

- Minimize using your arms and attempt not to use a rocking motion to assist you in getting up.

- Focus the tension on your leg and core muscles to get up.

- This exercise will help you stand and sit more easily since you train the motion, and it strengthens your legs for unbreakable stability.

Seated Leg Lift

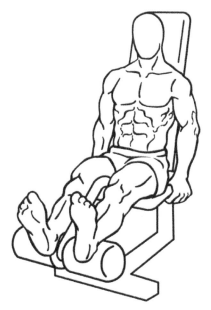

36. This exercise is great for building strength and increasing flexibility. Source: Everkinetic, CC BY-SA 3.0 <https://creativecommons.org/licenses/by-sa/3.0>, via Wikimedia Commons: https://commons.wikimedia.org/wiki/File:Seated-leg-curl-2.png

- Sit in a comfortable and solid chair, looking ahead with your back straight.

- Keep both feet flat on the ground, hip-width apart.

- Slowly lift your right leg, bending your knee toward your chest.

- You can use your arms to pull your leg up if you need additional assistance.

- Keep your leg pressed as close to your chest as it can reach.

- Hold your leg in this position for about five seconds before slowly lowering it.

- Repeat this motion five times with each leg.

- You will feel the tension in your hamstrings and glutes and the tendons in your knees being worked.

- This exercise is great for building strength and increasing flexibility.

Seated Knee Extensions

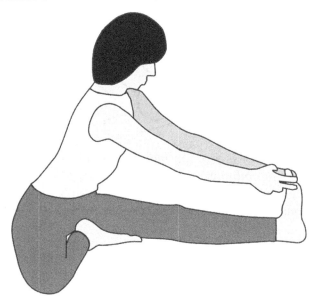

37. To complete a seated knee extension, sit straight up on a comfortable chair. Source: https://pixabay.com/vectors/yoga-woman-exercising-exercises-37267/

- To complete a seated knee extension, sit straight up on a comfortable chair.

- Extend one leg out straight in front of you and pull your toes back to stretch your calf muscle and tense your thighs.

- Your leg should be extended with your heel facing the floor and your toes pointing at the ceiling.

- Hold this position for five seconds before slowly lowering your leg.

- Ensure the tension is not released too quickly, which could cause injury.

- Repeat this exercise five to ten times for each leg.

Ankle Pumps

- To complete an ankle pump, you will first do a seated knee extension as described in the previous exercise.

- Point your toes forward, hold the position for five seconds, then point your toes to the ceiling, holding the position for five seconds.

- Cycle through the movements about three to five times before switching legs and repeating the exercise.

- You can finish the set by lifting both legs and doing the same thing with both feet.

- This activity works your upper and lower legs to get your muscles in unison for balancing.

Knee Extensions

Wall Slides

Sometimes, a squat can be extremely difficult, especially if your mobility has been affected by the aging process. A wall slide can be an alternative because a wall provides support to perform a squat motion. Many people do not begin the journey of improving themselves because they fear they cannot do complex exercises. Workouts like wall slides are superb for people who want to push themselves but also need security to ensure that they do not get injured. Using the environment around you to increase your balance lets you transform your space into an elite gym, and your results will be incredible.

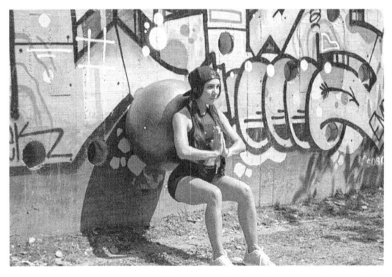

38. The aim is to get your thighs parallel to the ground, but if you cannot go that low, stop where you can. Source: Tyler Read, CC BY 2.0 <https://creativecommons.org/licenses/by/2.0>, via Wikimedia Commons: https://commons.wikimedia.org/wiki/File:Stability_ball_squats_o utdoors.jpg

- Stand with your back against the wall and slowly slide down.

- The aim is to get your thighs parallel to the ground, but if you cannot go that low, stop where you can.

- You can use the wall for grip using your arms to assist the motion down and up.

- This exercise is of greater difficulty than the other activities listed, so you should work your way up to it or be confident you can complete it.

- Ten repetitions of this exercise are more than enough to give yourself a great leg workout and get your joints into prime condition, too.

Hamstring Curls

Hamstring curls are a fun workout with minimal danger because you do them lying down.

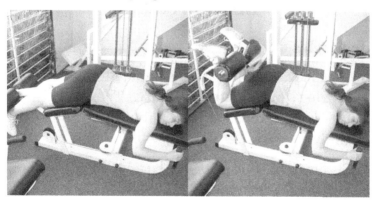

39. Hamstring curls are a fun workout with minimal danger because you do them lying down. Source: No machine-readable author provided. GeorgeStepanek assumed (based on copyright claims)., CC BY-SA 3.0 <http://creativecommons.org/licenses/by-sa/3.0/>, via Wikimedia Commons: https://commons.wikimedia.org/wiki/File:LyingLegCurlMachineE xercise.JPG

- Lie flat on your stomach and place a foam roller, a towel, or a firm pillow under your ankles.

- Lift your legs off the floor as you get comfortable on your belly.

- Complete about ten to twenty repetitions of this exercise.

- Be slow and deliberate with your movements, and do not allow your legs to collapse back onto the foam roller.

- Rather, place your legs slowly down because this has the double-sided benefit of minimizing the risk of injury and keeping the prolonged tension on the muscles to increase the exercise's effectiveness in strengthening the leg muscles.

Ankle Stretching

Ankle Circles

Strong ankles significantly contribute to remaining stable while moving and when sedentary. Therefore, the right stretches and exercises can improve your balance significantly.

- Sit down on a chair or the edge of your bed with your feet flat on the floor.

- Lift your right leg, extending it forward.

- You can use your arms to assist in lifting your leg as you stretch your leg.

- Rotate your ankle to the right slowly five times, then rotate it to the left slowly five times.

- Switch legs and do the same for your left ankle.

- Repeat the exercise for twenty rotations, ten clockwise and ten counter-clockwise.

- Ankle circles strengthen your tendons and muscles, creating the flexibility for improved balance.

Achilles Stretch

- As the name suggests, The Achilles stretch works on the Achilles tendon and the muscles surrounding that part of the ankle.

- This deep stretch can provide almost instant relief from ankle and foot pain.

- Use a chair or walker to balance on or lean against the wall.

- Extend your arms out in front of you using your chair to support your body weight.

- Step forward with your right leg, bending your knee slightly in a lunge-like position.

- Lean forward, keeping both heels on the ground.

- Switch between legs and experience the relief of this powerful stretch.

- Repeat the process about three times.

- This stretch will help you walk better by loosening the complex mix of sensitive tendons and bones in your feet and ankles.

Finding What Works for You

You know your body better than anyone else. The advice you receive from your doctor and your inner experiences should guide the exercise you choose. The above exercises are simple and easy to introduce into a daily routine. You have strengths and weaknesses, so you know which parts of your body desperately need the work. Therefore, you can mix and match each activity, tailoring them to your unique physique, lifestyle, and capabilities. Remember, the aim is not to compare yourself to the next person who may be progressing faster or performing the exercises better. You are running your race and seeking to surpass your past self.

Experiment with these different activities, especially in the beginning, and see where you get the most results. Furthermore, you can draft a schedule to break up the exercise into different muscle groups so you have time to rest certain parts of your body. Remember, if you are over 65 you require thirty minutes of exercise at least five days a week. Your exercise regime can be filled to the brim with many fun balancing activities. You can combine more cardio-heavy workouts with strength training and stretching so that your body gets everything it needs from a physical engagement perspective. Your health journey and balance exercise implementations should be put together like a personalized puzzle that fits exactly what you need at the moment. As you grow and improve you can make changes to suit your new capabilities to constantly put in the work that raises your quality of life.

Chapter 5: Strength and Stability

Your core, which runs from the bottom of your ribs to your buttocks, is crucial for balance and stability. It includes the belly, side muscles (obliques), and back muscles. These muscles help with everyday activities like getting out of bed, sitting, standing, and bending. They support your back, arms, and legs and need regular exercise to stay strong. Furthermore, a strong and stable core can prevent back pain.

Usually, sit-ups and crunches are the go-to exercises for a strong core. They aim to give you a flat stomach and a strong core. However, these exercises can strain your neck and back as you age. They pull your neck and press your spine against a hard surface, which isn't good for your back. Conditions like degenerative disc disease, back problems, and arthritis can make sit-ups and crunches painful and difficult to perform. These exercises mainly target the hip flexors, the muscles running from your lower back to your thighs. Overworking these muscles can cause lower back pain and discomfort.

A strong core is your safeguard against slips, trips, and mishaps when you're active, during sports, or any activity. A firm and flexible core provides support for nearly everything you do. Weak core muscles can lead to injuries, increased fatigue, reduced endurance, worsening lower back pain, posture problems, and muscle injuries. However, strengthening your core can have the opposite effect, potentially reducing back discomfort and the risk of falls.

Core exercises involve movements that engage your back and stomach muscles in coordination. These exercises aim to fortify the numerous large and small muscles that stabilize and support your pelvis and spine, making them more resilient. This improved strength enables better control of your pelvis and spine when they encounter external forces during physical activities and daily routines. Additionally, these areas are the foundation for all your movements and actions, stabilizing your spinal column, hips, and pelvic region. Consequently, you'll call upon your core muscles whenever you require support in any movement.

The exercises listed in this chapter include seated, standing, and floor-based options. As with any exercise routine, start slowly and progress to more challenging exercises over time. If you're uncertain about the suitability of a particular exercise for your needs, consulting your physician or a physiotherapist is advisable.

1. Abdominal Bracing

Abdominal bracing is a straightforward core exercise that offers substantial benefits for strength and stability, making it particularly helpful for older people. This exercise enhances posture, strengthens the core, and helps maintain an upright position, ultimately promoting better balance and overall well-being.

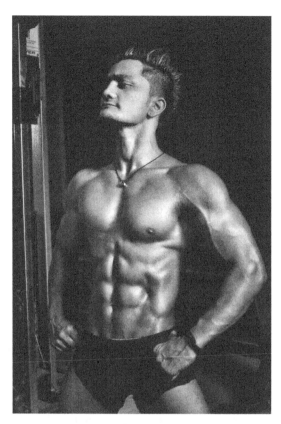

40. Abdominal bracing is a straightforward core exercise that offers substantial benefits for strength and stability. Source: https://www.pexels.com/photo/grayscale-photography-of-man-in-short-standiung-896059/

Instructions

1. Stand or sit up straight, ensuring you maintain good posture. Keep your shoulders relaxed and pulled back, preventing slouching.

2. As you maintain your upright posture, gently draw your belly button inward toward your spine. You should feel your abdominal muscles engage and provide support to your midsection.

3. Keep your belly button pulled in for as long as possible while continuing to breathe naturally. Avoid holding your breath during the exercise.

4. Perform this exercise multiple times throughout the day. Start with brief intervals and gradually increase the duration as you become more comfortable.

If you find this exercise challenging, consider the following modified version:

1. Sit comfortably in a chair with your feet flat on the floor. Ensure that your back is supported by the chair's backrest.

2. Sit straight and gently draw your belly button toward your spine, as in the standard version. Your abdominal muscles should engage and provide support.

3. Maintain the bracing of your core for as long as possible while breathing normally. Avoid holding your breath during the exercise.

Perform this seated version multiple times throughout the day, gradually increasing the duration as you become more at ease with the exercise.

2. Knee Lifts

Knee lifts are a simple and effective exercise promoting lower body strength and stability, making it ideal for older individuals. Incorporating this exercise into your routine can enhance your leg muscles, improve balance, and contribute to overall well-being.

Instructions

1. Begin by sitting in a sturdy chair with your feet resting firmly on the ground. Make sure that you're sitting slightly forward and your back does not touch the chair's backrest. This encourages an upright posture and engages your core.

2. To maintain stability, you can grip the sides of the chair with your hands.

3. Lift one leg a few inches off the ground while continuing to engage your core muscles. This action helps with balance and strengthens your lower body. Hold this raised position for about five seconds.

4. Lower the lifted leg back to the ground, keeping your back straight. Then, repeat the lifting and holding action with the other leg.

5. Perform this exercise ten times for each leg. As you become more comfortable, you can gradually increase the number of repetitions.

If you find the standard knee lifts challenging, you can try a seated modification:

1. Sit comfortably in a chair with your feet flat on the floor. This time your back can be supported by the chair's backrest.

2. Lift one leg a few inches off the ground while keeping your core engaged. Hold this position for about five seconds.

3. Lower the lifted leg back to the ground, ensuring your back remains against the chair's backrest. Then, repeat the same lifting and holding action with the other leg.

Perform this seated version ten times for each leg, gradually increasing the repetitions as you gain confidence.

---

3. Leg Lifts

Leg lifts offer an excellent way to simultaneously engage and strengthen your abdominal and oblique muscles. You have the choice of performing them while sitting or lying down, depending on your preference. If you're new to this exercise, it's recommended to begin in a chair and progress to the lying-down version. Leg lifts help you build a strong core and enhance stability.

Instructions

1. Seated Leg Lifts (Beginners):

1. Sit up straight in a sturdy chair with your feet firmly on the floor.

2. Pay attention to your core muscles.

3. Lift your left foot as high as possible while maintaining good posture and a straight back. Hold this raised position for several seconds.

4. Slowly release your leg and place it back on the floor.

5. Perform the same movement with your right leg.

2. Lying Down Leg Lifts:

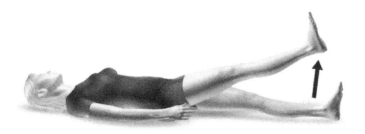

Straight Leg Raise

41. Beginners often begin with seated leg lifts, and as they gain confidence and strength, they progress to the lying-down version. Source: BruceBlaus, CC BY-SA 4.0 <https://creativecommons.org/licenses/by-sa/4.0>, via Wikimedia Commons: https://commons.wikimedia.org/wiki/File:Exercise_Straight_Leg _Raises.png

1. Lie flat on your back with your arms resting at your sides.

2. Engage your core muscles.

3. Raise your left leg a few inches off the floor. Hold this elevated position for a brief moment.

4. Slowly release your leg and let it return to the floor.

5. Repeat the exercise with your right leg.

Note: You can choose the variation that best suits your fitness and comfort. Beginners often begin with seated leg lifts, and as they gain confidence and strength, they progress to the lying-down version.

---

4. Leg Taps

Leg taps are a beneficial exercise to improve lower body strength, flexibility, and core stability. This exercise can be performed while sitting in a chair, making it accessible for everyone, especially older adults.

Instructions

1. Sit in a sturdy chair with your feet flat on the ground.

2. Ensure you maintain an upright posture by sitting forward on the chair and your back straight, not leaning against the backrest.

3. You can hold onto the bottom of your seat for added support if needed.

4. Activate your abdominal muscles by drawing your belly button inward toward your spine.

5. Extend both legs in front of you. Keep your legs straight but not locked.

6. Gently tap the floor with both feet five times. This movement engages your leg muscles and promotes flexibility.

7. Slowly bend your knees, moving your feet back toward the chair.

8. Repeat the exercise ten times, taking a few seconds to rest.

Regular leg taps will improve lower body strength, flexibility, and core stability. This exercise is accessible and can be easily incorporated into your daily routine for enhanced well-being and physical fitness.

5. Seated Side Bends

Seated side bends are a great way to strengthen your internal and external oblique and abdominal muscles. This exercise can be performed comfortably in a chair and is perfect for people looking to enhance their core strength.

Instructions

1. Sit comfortably in a sturdy chair with your knees bent and feet flat on the ground. Ensure that your posture is upright.

2. Place the palm of your left hand behind your head. Extend your left elbow, aligning it with your ear.

3. Keep your right arm at your side, in line with your upper torso.

4. Inhale and exhale naturally, maintaining a straight and upright posture.

5. Begin by tilting your body to the right, bringing your right arm closer to the floor. Simultaneously, pull back your left elbow. This movement creates a stretch on the left side of your torso.

6. Hold this stretched position for a moment.

7. Slowly return to an upright seated position. Transition to the opposite side and repeat the exercise by stretching the right side.

8. Perform this side bend exercise ten times on each side.

This exercise targets and strengthens your oblique and abdominal muscles. It helps enhance your core strength.

6. Wood Chops

Wood chops are a versatile exercise that can be performed sitting or standing, offering a dynamic way to engage multiple muscle groups. This exercise enhances core strength, improves balance, and increases flexibility. It's suitable for people wanting to add variety to their routine and promote overall fitness.

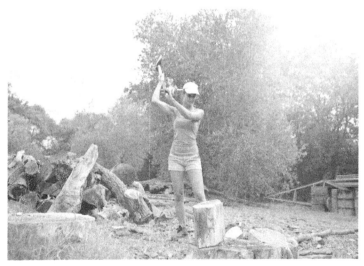

42. Wood chops are a versatile exercise that can be performed sitting or standing, offering a dynamic way to engage multiple muscle groups. Source: https://www.pexels.com/photo/young-woman-chopping-wood-in-countryside-3769731/

Instructions

1. Decide whether you want to perform this exercise sitting or standing. Use a sturdy chair with your feet flat on the floor if sitting. If standing, ensure your back is straight, and your feet are shoulder-width apart.

2. Start by placing your hands together and holding your arms straight out in front of you.

3. Use a lightweight object, like a water bottle, to add resistance during the movement.

4. Begin by raising your hands to your left shoulder.

5. Then, swing (or chop) your arms down toward your right hip while keeping your body straight.

6. Repeat this chopping action ten times, aiming for a fluid motion.

7. Bring your hands back to your left shoulder after completing the right-to-left chop.

8. Continue the exercise by moving between your right shoulder and left hip, repeating the same chopping motion.

9. Initially, focus on using only your arms and maintaining a straight back and body.

10. As you become more comfortable, add a twist to your body toward the downward chop as you move your arms, intensifying the exercise.

Practicing wood chops, whether seated or standing, strengthens your core, improves balance, and enhances flexibility.

7. Seated Forward Roll-Ups

Seated forward roll-ups focus on strengthening the upper and lower abdominal muscles. This exercise can be done while sitting in a chair, making it accessible and ideal to enhance your core strength.

Instructions

1. Sit up straight in your chair.

2. Extend your legs in front of you, with your toes pointing upward and your heels resting on the floor.

3. Keep your arms extended in front of you while maintaining good posture and a straight back.

4. Roll your upper body forward by pushing your hands toward the opposite wall and guiding your chest closer to your legs.

5. Maintain this position for a few seconds, feeling the stretch in your core muscles.

6. Gradually straighten your back and rise to a seated position again.

7. Take a few seconds to rest before repeating the exercise.

8. Aim to complete a total of 10 repetitions.

This exercise requires slow and gentle movements to ensure its effectiveness. Avoid relying on your shoulders or back for momentum. The goal is to engage your core muscles.

8. Dead Bug

The Dead Bug exercise may appear complex at first, but it's a remarkable method to target and strengthen your core while seated. This variation is especially helpful for those focusing on core improvement. It helps enhance core stability, balance, and coordination.

Instructions

1. Begin by sitting on a sturdy, straight-back chair.

2. Lean back in the chair, allowing your feet to rest on the ground and your arms resting on your thighs.

3. Place a pillow or cushion behind your back to help maintain a straight spine during this exercise.

4. Engage your core muscles.

5. Raise the opposing arm overhead and reach toward the ceiling while you extend one leg straight out, parallel to the floor.

6. Keep your head up and keep your focus in front of you.

7. Hold this position for 10 or so seconds.

8. Slowly return to the starting position.

9. Use the opposing arm and leg to repeat this exercise on the other side.

Advanced Variation (without Back Support)

- For an added challenge, this exercise can be performed without the back support, further engaging your core muscles.

Note: The Dead Bug exercise can also be done while lying on your back, extending opposing arms and legs toward the ceiling.

---

9. Sit to Stand

The Sit to Stand exercise is a fundamental movement that helps enhance lower body strength and overall stability. It's especially valuable for improving your ability to stand up from a seated position.

Instructions

1. Start by sitting in a chair with a firm, hard surface.

2. For beginners, using a chair with armrests to assist you in standing up is advisable.

3. As you progress, you can transition to using only one armrest or no armrests.

4. You can place your hands crossed on your chest for a more advanced variation to engage your core further.

5. Ensure your feet are flat on the floor.

6. Tighten your abdominal muscles.

7. Lean forward slightly. Use the strength of your leg muscles to stand up from the chair.

8. Avoid pushing up with your arms if you use the chair's armrests for support. Rely on your leg muscles.

9. Stand for a few seconds with your back straight.

---

10. Engage your core muscles as you gently lean your body forward and lower yourself back into the chair.

11. Repeat this exercise ten times.

By consistently practicing the sit-to-stand exercise, you'll improve your lower body strength and ability to transition from seated to standing.

---

10. Bird-Dog

The Quadruped, or the Bird-Dog exercise, is a powerful way to enhance core strength, balance, and coordination. It targets multiple muscle groups, making it a versatile addition to your routine.

Note: This exercise may be challenging for individuals with knee issues. Proceed cautiously, and consider placing a pillow or a towel beneath your knees for added comfort and support.

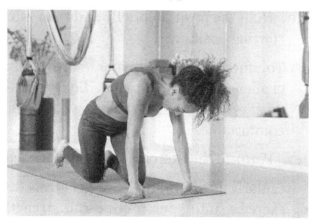

43. The Quadruped, or the Bird-Dog exercise, is a powerful way to enhance core strength, balance, and coordination. Source: https://www.pexels.com/photo/woman-exercising-indoors-6582970/

Instructions

1. Begin by getting down on your hands and knees.

2. Ensure your hands are directly under your shoulders and your knees are beneath your hips.

3. Gaze at the ground to maintain a neutral neck position.

4. Tighten your core muscles to stabilize your spine.

5. Simultaneously, extend your left arm and right leg until they are parallel to the floor.

6. This movement is executed by contracting your core muscles to maintain balance.

7. Maintain this extended position for a moment.

8. Carefully lower your extended arm and leg back to the ground.

9. Now, extend your right arm and left leg in the same manner.

10. Hold the position briefly and then return to the starting position.

11. To further engage your core muscles and challenge your stability, hold the extended position for 30 seconds as you become more comfortable.

12. Perform the exercise ten times for each side.

Regularly incorporating the Quadruped, or Bird-Dog exercise, into your routine can strengthen your core, improve balance, and enhance overall coordination. This exercise can be adapted to your fitness level and is a valuable addition to your daily workout regimen.

11. Plank

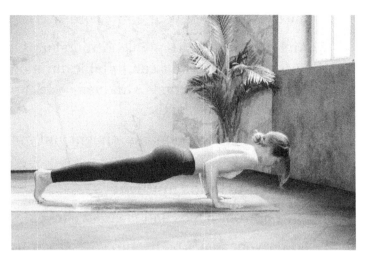

44. *The plank is a classic core-strengthening exercise that engages your core muscles simultaneously, providing remarkable benefits despite its apparent simplicity. Source: https://www.pexels.com/photo/woman-in-black-tank-top-and-black-leggings-doing-yoga-3823063/*

The plank is a classic core-strengthening exercise that engages your core muscles simultaneously, providing remarkable benefits despite its apparent simplicity. It's known for its effectiveness, especially for people over 50, and helps boost core strength and stability.

Instructions

Traditional Forearm Plank (Floor)

1. Begin by lying flat on the ground with your hands positioned near your shoulders, similar to a push-up position.

2. Lift yourself up by pressing into your forearms while keeping your feet on the floor. Maintain a straight back and engage your core muscles.

3. Press down with your elbows and forearms. Contract your glutes, quadriceps, and abdominal muscles to engage your entire core.

4. Aim to maintain this plank position for as long as possible. Begin with a comfortable duration, even if it's only a few seconds. Gradually work up to 10, 20, or even 30 seconds.

5. Ensure your back remains straight and your core tight throughout the exercise.

Modified Plank (on Hands and Knees)

1. Start on your hands and knees as above.

2. Lower your upper body onto your forearms, with your shoulders directly on top of your elbows.

3. Maintain a straight back and hip alignment. Keep your knees on the ground with your feet in the air.

Wall Plank (Alternative)

1. If the traditional plank is challenging, consider a wall plank. Place your forearms against a wall.

2. Step back slightly to create a slight angle with your body.

3. Maintain a straight back and hip alignment. Keep your forearms flat against the wall.

4. Hold this position for as long as you can comfortably manage.

Note: Gradually increasing the duration while maintaining proper form is key to reaping the full benefits of this exercise.

Whether performed on the floor or with modifications, the plank is an excellent exercise to enhance core strength and stability. It can be tailored to your fitness level and is a valuable addition to your daily exercise routine.

12. The Bridge

The Bridge is a challenging core exercise requiring some flexibility. It's a fantastic method for working your core and developing strength and flexibility.

Traditional Bridge (Floor)

1. Begin by lying with your back flat on the ground, your knees bent, and your feet on the floor.

2. Engage your core muscles.

3. Lift your hips off the ground, creating a straight line from your chest to your knees. Hold this position while taking three breaths.

4. Ensure your back is straight and not curved. Release the pose, lower your hips, and repeat the exercise a few more times.

Bridge with Exercise Ball (Advanced)

Note: This variation requires an exercise ball and is best performed with a partner to assist with stability.

1. Sit carefully on a large exercise ball with your feet on the floor. Keep your knees at a 90-degree angle.

2. Roll your body toward your knees so that the ball supports your shoulders and head. Your core should be engaged throughout this movement.

3. Press your hips toward the ceiling while maintaining a 90-degree angle at your knees.

Only your shoulders and head should be resting on the exercise ball.

By incorporating the Bridge exercise on the floor or using an exercise ball, you can effectively target your core muscles and enhance strength and flexibility. This exercise can be tailored to your fitness level and is a valuable addition to your regular exercise routine.

Chapter 6: Flexibility and Mobility

Undeniably, aging affects a person's mobility and is an entirely natural part of life. As you age, your joints and tendons weaken, significantly impacting your ability to move freely. However, there is hope in the form of exercises like stretching, which can improve joint flexibility. This newfound flexibility allows a range of movements, from easier neck and back actions to more effortless hip and thigh movements and arm mobility.

For instance, think about when you found it challenging to turn your head or bend to pick up something due to stiffness. This is a common experience among many seniors. Flexibility exercises like stretching combat these limitations and enhance mobility, making everyday life in your golden years more enjoyable and manageable.

These exercises address various key areas, like neck and back movements. By focusing on these muscle groups, stretching can alleviate discomfort and reduce stiffness. Imagine being able to turn your head easily, enhancing the pleasure of a simple walk, or even just looking around the room. Your range of motion extends to your hips and thighs.

Strong and flexible hips and thighs are essential for everyday activities like getting in and out of chairs, cars, or beds. Regular stretching makes these movements smoother and less strenuous.

Your arms and shoulders will also benefit from stretching exercises. Enhanced flexibility means reaching for objects on high shelves, lifting items, and performing everyday tasks with less difficulty, ensuring independence.

These flexibility exercises become invaluable tools in your daily life. You'll notice improvements in various routine activities. For example, dressing becomes more manageable as you can reach your feet to put on shoes and socks or fasten buttons and zippers without straining your arms and shoulders. If you're a gardening enthusiast, stretching can make bending, kneeling, and reaching for your favorite plants less taxing. Similarly, you'll find preparing meals easier in the kitchen, from reaching for ingredients to stirring pots and even playing with your grandchildren, whether playing catch or helping them with their shoelaces becomes less of a challenge with improved mobility.

This chapter covers every flexibility exercise you would need. In addition to basic stretching techniques, you can regularly practice yoga or tai chi to work on your mobility. However, keep a few essential tips in mind. Start with a brief warm-up before you begin your flexibility exercises. This warms up your muscles and prepares them for stretching. When stretching, aim to hold each position for about 10 to 20 seconds to allow your muscles to relax and extend gradually.

Always remember stretching should never cause pain. If you feel discomfort, it's best to avoid that particular stretch. Deep breathing is your ally during these exercises. Taking a deep breath and slowly exhaling as you stretch can help relax your body and deepen your stretches. Finally, keep a chair close by while you exercise for added safety and support. It can provide stability and assistance if needed.

---

1. Overhead Shoulder Mobility

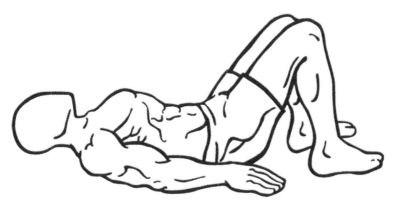

45. The overhead shoulder mobility stretch is essential for improving the flexibility and range of motion in your shoulders and upper back. Source: Everkinetic, CC BY-SA 3.0 <https://creativecommons.org/licenses/by-sa/3.0>, via Wikimedia Commons: https://commons.wikimedia.org/wiki/File:Bridge-2.png

The overhead shoulder mobility stretch is essential for improving the flexibility and range of motion in your shoulders and upper back. This exercise targets the latissimus dorsi muscles, crucial for various daily activities and maintaining good posture. It also helps alleviate tension in the upper back and promotes a more relaxed and upright posture.

Instructions

1. Begin by lying flat on the ground with your knees bent and your feet flat on the floor. Your arms should be at your sides.

2. Slowly raise your arms while keeping your shoulders in contact with the ground. Your palms should be facing up.

3. Lower your right arm toward the floor behind you, extending it over your head, keeping it straight. The goal is to reach the ground with your hand without lifting your back.

4. Hold the stretched position for 10 to 20 seconds, feeling the stretch in your legs and shoulders.

5. Return your right arm to the upright position, then repeat the stretch with your left arm.

6. Perform this stretch three to four times with each arm.

Modified Version

1. Start in the same position, lying flat on the ground with your knees bent and feet flat.

2. Instead of attempting to touch the ground with your hand, focus on gently extending your arms over your head without any strain.

3. Hold the stretch for about 10 seconds, then return your arms to the starting position.

4. Perform this modified stretch three to four times with each arm.

5. As you become more comfortable, gradually work toward touching the ground, but ensure you never push yourself into discomfort.

Understanding the Results

If your back lifts off the ground while attempting this stretch, it indicates a need for improved shoulder and lat flexibility. This could be due to tightness in the lats. On the other hand, if your back remains on the ground, but you still can't touch the floor with your arm, it points to a lack of shoulder mobility. By practicing this stretch regularly, you can address these issues and enhance your overhead shoulder mobility.

2. Ankle Dorsiflexion

Ankle dorsiflexion is crucial for maintaining proper alignment of the lower limbs and for activities like walking, squatting, and going up or down stairs. This exercise targets the flexibility and mobility of the ankle joint and helps improve your overall lower body function.

Instructions

1. Begin by placing your front leg at a 90-degree angle, with your foot flat on the floor and toes facing the wall.

2. Lower yourself into a half-kneeling position, ensuring your back leg is also bent at a 90-degree angle with the foot flat on the ground.

3. The toes of your front foot should be about 4 inches away from the wall.

4. Gradually move your body forward until your front knee directly faces the wall. Keep your foot flat on the ground throughout the movement.

5. Attempt to make contact between your knee and the wall while maintaining a flat foot.

6. You can use your hands to push against the wall to assist in this movement gently. Ensure your knee passes directly over your foot.

7. Repeat this process for a few attempts with your current leg.

8. Repeat the same steps with the opposite leg to evaluate the mobility of the other ankle.

Understanding the Results

It is a positive sign of reasonable ankle mobility if you can touch your knee to the wall while keeping your foot flat on the ground. This exercise helps identify and address limitations in ankle dorsiflexion. If reaching the wall is challenging, regular practice can improve your ankle flexibility and overall lower body function.

---

3. Spinal Flexion and Extension

Spinal flexion and extension are vital for maintaining a healthy and flexible spine. These movements help alleviate tension, improve posture, and enhance overall mobility in your back. This exercise targets your entire spine, from your neck to your lower back, promoting a greater range of motion.

Instructions

1. Begin by positioning yourself on your hands and knees, with your legs hip-distance apart and your hands beneath your shoulders.

2. Start with the "cat-cow" sequence. For spinal flexion (the "cow" position), press through your hands while raising your shoulders, rounding your upper back, and pulling the shoulders apart.

Simultaneously, tuck your chin toward your chest.

3. Hold the spinal flexion position for a moment, focusing on the stretch along your back.

4. Transition to spinal extension (the "cat" position) by raising your head and bringing your shoulder blades together. Slowly bring your spine back to a neutral position.

5. Then, push your chest down and arch your back, bringing your shoulder blades together. This is the spinal extension.

6. Perform the cat-cow sequence for 10 to 20 seconds, focusing on smooth and controlled movements.

7. Repeat the sequence several times, allowing your spine to flex and extend.

Understanding the Results

This exercise evaluates your spinal flexibility. If you cannot fully extend or flex your spine, it suggests a need for mobility stretches. Regular practice of the cat-cow sequence will help improve the flexibility of your spine, reduce stiffness, and promote a healthier, more mobile back. It's an excellent addition to your routine to enhance your overall spinal health and mobility.

---

4. Thoracic Rotation

Thoracic rotation is essential for maintaining flexibility and mobility in the upper and middle back. It helps prevent stiffness and enhances your ability to perform rotational movements, which are crucial for various activities in daily life. This exercise targets the thoracic spine and helps assess and improve your spine's rotational mobility.

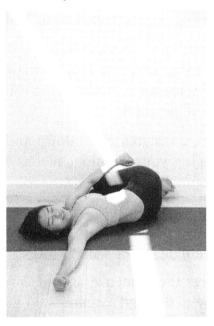

46. Thoracic rotation is essential for maintaining flexibility and mobility in the upper and middle back. Source: https://www.pexels.com/photo/fit-asian-woman-doing-supine-spinal-twist-on-yoga-mat-7592444/

Instructions

1. Start by kneeling and place a thick towel, a few books, or a yoga block between your knees to provide resistance and support for your legs.

2. Sit back on your heels while creating an inward squeeze with your thighs against the yoga block or object of choice.

3. If kneeling in this posture causes discomfort in your knees or ankles, an alternative is to perform it seated in a chair.

4. Extend your left hand to your right shoulder and your right hand to your left shoulder, passing your right hand underneath your left arm.

5. Rotate your upper body toward the right side as far as possible. Maintain contact between your hands at your shoulders and ensure your elbows are roughly at shoulder height.

6. Slowly return to the middle position, then rotate to the right side again. Repeat this rotation a few more times, attempting to go farther each time.

7. Keep your hips and legs aligned to the front as you perform the rotation. The focus is on the upper and middle back, not the lower back.

8. Maintain squared hips by pressing your thighs against the block or maintaining proper posture in the chair.

9. After completing the rotations on one side, switch to the other side by placing your right hand beneath your left arm and tilting your body to the left.

Understanding the Results

This exercise evaluates your thoracic rotation mobility. If you achieve less than 45 degrees of rotation, it indicates that your spine mobility needs improvement. A rotation of 45 degrees or more suggests good mobility. Regularly practicing this exercise can help increase your thoracic rotation, reduce upper and middle back stiffness, and enhance spine mobility.

5. Hip Flexion

Hip flexion is crucial for various activities, from walking to climbing stairs. This exercise focuses on assessing and improving your hip flexibility and mobility. It targets the muscles responsible for raising your legs and aids in preventing stiffness and discomfort.

Instructions

1. Start by lying on your back with your legs fully extended.

2. Place your arms out to the sides with your palms facing down, and engage your lower abdomen by bracing it.

3. Press your hands firmly into the ground to stabilize your upper body.

4. Begin by flexing your right knee and drawing it as close to your chest as possible while keeping your left leg as straight as you can.

5. Then, raise your right leg toward your upper torso while maintaining a flat back. This movement should be controlled and gradual.

6. Hold your raised leg in this position for 10 to 20 seconds to feel the stretch in your hip flexor.

7. Slowly lower your right leg to the starting position.

8. Repeat the same process with your left leg, drawing it as close to your chest as possible and raising it toward your upper torso.

9. Perform this exercise with both legs for a few repetitions.

Understanding the Results

The goal of this exercise is to evaluate your hip flexion mobility. If you can raise your heel past your knee on the bottom leg, it indicates reasonable mobility. An ideal range of motion is reached when you can raise your leg to 90 degrees, with your legs perpendicular to each other. It indicates your hip flexors are flexible, and your range of motion is ideal. If it is challenging to reach 90 degrees, regular practice of this exercise can help improve your hip flexibility and mobility, making everyday activities more comfortable and efficient.

---

6. Whole Body Stretch

This advanced stretch offers a comprehensive whole-body stretch for individuals with good mobility and balance. It targets multiple muscle groups, promoting flexibility and balance. The exercise encompasses various movements to enhance overall body mobility.

Instructions

1. Begin by stepping your right leg forward into a low lunge position. Your left leg should be extended straight behind you.

2. Lower yourself into the low lunge, ensuring your right knee is positioned directly above your right ankle.

3. Place your hands on either side of your front foot for stability.

4. Move your right elbow inward, positioning it near your right foot.

5. Keep your back flat and focus on squaring your hips forward to create balance and stability.

6. Rotate your upper body to the right and extend your right arm upward. This movement involves the thoracic spine.

7. While doing this, maintain square hips as much as possible, emphasizing the twist in your upper body.

8. Reverse the motion once you've reached a comfortable twist with your arm extended.

9. Extend your right leg from this position to achieve a hamstring stretch. As you do, round your upper back for spinal flexion.

10. To return your right leg to the downward dog posture, push through your hands and bring your right leg back.

11. Step your left leg forward and repeat the entire sequence on the other side.

Understanding the Results

This advanced whole-body stretch enhances your overall mobility and flexibility. Regular practice can help improve balance, spinal flexibility, and lower body flexibility. If you're capable of performing this sequence easily, it indicates good mobility and balance. However, if it is challenging, continue practicing to achieve better mobility and balance throughout your body.

7. Chair Yoga

Regular yoga practice has been proven to enhance overall well-being, but it's essential to recognize that yoga can be adapted to accommodate individuals with varying ability levels. Chair yoga is a wonderful option incorporating a range of postures to improve balance focus and reduce joint strain. It's an accessible and inclusive way to experience the benefits of yoga, making it suitable for individuals with physical limitations, those who find traditional yoga challenging, and those who struggle with balance or getting on and off the floor.

Instructions

1. Seated Mountain Pose

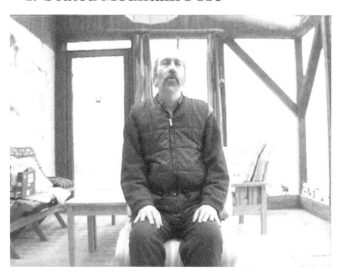

47. Regular yoga practice has been proven to enhance overall well-being. Source: Nobody60, CC BY-SA 3.0 <https://creativecommons.org/licenses/by-sa/3.0>, via Wikimedia Commons: https://commons.wikimedia.org/wiki/File:8.F%C3%BC%C3%9Fe_ bewegen.png

1. Sit on a chair with your feet flat on the floor and your back straight.

2. Rest your hands on your thighs or knees.

3. Take a few deep breaths and focus on your posture, feeling rooted and stable.

2. Seated Forward Fold

1. Sit at the front edge of your chair with feet hip-width apart.

2. Inhale, elongate your spine, and as you exhale, bend forward from your hips, folding forward.

3. Let your arms hang or rest your hands on your legs.

4. Breathe deeply and feel the stretch along your spine and hamstrings.

3. Seated Cat-Cow

1. Sit with feet flat on the floor.

2. Inhale, arch your back and look up (Cow Pose).

3. Exhale, round your back, and tuck your chin (Cat Pose).

4. Continue this gentle flow, coordinating your breath with the movements.

4. Seated Spinal Twist

1. Sit with your feet flat.

2. Inhale and lengthen your spine.

3. Exhale, twist to the right, holding the back of your chair with your hands.

4. Breathe deeply and feel the gentle twist along your spine.

5. Repeat on the left side.

5. Chair Warrior I

1. Sit with your feet flat.

2. Lift your right foot and place it on the chair.

3. Inhale, extend your arms upward and lengthen your spine.

4. Breathe deeply, focusing on stability and balance.

5. Repeat with the left foot on the chair.

6. Seated Relaxation

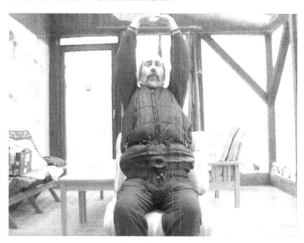

48. Chair yoga is a wonderful option incorporating a range of postures to improve balance focus and reduce joint strain. Source: Nobody60, CC BY-SA 3.0 <https://creativecommons.org/licenses/by-sa/3.0>, via Wikimedia Commons: https://commons.wikimedia.org/wiki/File:1.Ausstrecken.png

1. Sit comfortably in your chair with your eyes closed.

2. Focus on your breath, inhaling and exhaling deeply and slowly.

3. Let go of tension and enjoy a moment of relaxation.

Note: The key to chair yoga is adapting each posture to your needs. Always prioritize safety and comfort.

---

8. Tai Chi

If you are seeking a method to alleviate tension, strengthen your body, and enhance your balance, consider tai chi. Initially developed for self-defense, tai chi has evolved into an elegant exercise renowned for its stress relief and various health benefits. This practice, often described as "meditation in motion," consists of flowing, graceful movements promoting physical and mental well-being.

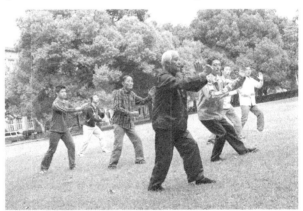

49. Tai chi has evolved into an elegant exercise renowned for its stress relief and various health benefits. Source: Seattletaijiquan, CC BY-SA 4.0 <https://creativecommons.org/licenses/by-sa/4.0>, via Wikimedia Commons: https://commons.wikimedia.org/wiki/File:Tai_Chi_Chuan_In_The_Park.jpg

Instructions

1. Begin with a gentle warm-up to prepare your body. You can start by standing with your feet hip-width apart and doing light stretching and deep breathing. Relax and clear your mind.

2. Stand with your feet shoulder-width apart, knees slightly bent, and your weight evenly distributed between both legs. Keep your back straight, shoulders relaxed, and your head held high.

3. Focus on your breath. Breathe gently out through your mouth after taking a deep breath through your nose that causes your abdomen to expand. During the practice, maintain a rhythmic and natural breathing pattern.

4. Tai chi consists of a series of slow, flowing movements. Here's a simple sequence to get you started:

   1. Opening: Begin with your hands at your sides, palms facing inwards.

   2. Ward Off: Step your left foot forward and simultaneously move your hands, creating a circular motion.

   3. Rollback: Shift your weight back onto your right leg and turn your hands.

   4. Press: Shift your weight forward and push your hands forward.

   5. Push: Continue pushing your hands forward while stepping forward with your right foot.

5. Tai chi emphasizes balance. Pay attention to the weight distribution between your legs in each movement and maintain a centered balance.

6. While performing tai chi, concentrate on the moment. Focus on your breath, the sensations in your body, and the movements. This meditative aspect is a key element of tai chi.

7. Conclude your tai chi practice by returning to the starting position. Stand with your feet shoulder-width apart, hands at your sides, and take a few deep breaths. Acknowledge the benefits of your practice and relax.

Regular physical activity is a cornerstone of healthy aging. It is well-established that any physical activity is better than none for improving mobility and overall health, particularly for seniors. A well-planned and monitored mobility workout can be a game-changer for seniors. These specially developed exercise routines are tailored to address the unique needs of older adults, focusing on enhancing mobility, strength, and balance.

Chapter 7: Progression and Tracking

Working on improving balance and mobility is undoubtedly an excellent endeavor to maintain an active and vibrant lifestyle. Still, have you thought about how you would know if you're making progress and enhancing your abilities with balance exercises? The answer is to track the progress.

Knowing where you stand and the improvements you've made provides insights that can be evaluated to tweak the exercise routine further and improve the outcomes. You can increase the intensity of exercises and overcome plateaus without a hitch. The information shared in this chapter will provide the proper guidance and motivate you to stay on your path toward a healthy life without balance issues.

Tracking Your Progress

Tracking progress in balance exercises is essential for several reasons. It serves as a powerful motivator. When you can see tangible improvements over time, it encourages you to stay committed and consistent with your exercise routine. Likewise, tracking provides accountability, holding you responsible for your fitness goals. It helps you identify areas needing more attention and refinement. You can also set clear, achievable goals by meticulously documenting your progress. These goals act as guiding beacons, giving you direction and purpose in your balance exercise journey.

Tracking progress allows necessary adjustments to your balance exercises. Ensuring your routines remain compelling and challenging as your abilities improve is crucial. Regular assessments and data tracking help you fine-tune your workouts to match your evolving capabilities. Beyond enhancing your fitness, monitoring progress is a valuable health monitoring tool. You will detect potential issues early and address them proactively by tracking changes. Whether you maintain a workout journal, set specific goals, conduct regular assessments, use technology, or seek professional guidance, tracking ensures your balance exercises are safe, efficient, and tailored to your needs and goals.

Here's what you must do and the methods to apply for maximum results.

Maintaining a Workout Journal

A workout journal is your compass in the world of balance exercises. It is a comprehensive record of your fitness journey, offering insights into your progress and areas needing improvement. Record the date of each balance exercise session for accurate tracking and reference. Specify the balance exercises you perform in detail, including their names and descriptions. Document how much time you dedicate to each exercise or how long you maintain specific positions.

Keep meticulous counts of the repetitions and sets for each exercise. You can add detailed comments about your workout experiences, and don't forget to include information about how you felt during the session, challenges encountered, and improvements noticed. Consider personalizing your workout journal with your thoughts and feelings. Use it as a fitness diary reflecting on your progress. Lastly, share your achievements, no matter how small, to stay motivated and celebrate your accomplishments.

Setting Clear Goals

Goals provide direction and purpose in your exercise routine to improve balance. They help you stay focused and motivated. When setting goals, ensure they are clear and well-defined. While setting objectives, avoid vague ideas or goals that still need clarification. For example, instead of setting a goal to get better control while walking, specify you want to enhance the balance duration for improved mobility. After establishing which goals to set, create concrete metrics to track progress. For example, set a goal to increase your balance duration by 10 seconds weekly.

You can set long-term goals, but the goals and objectives should be realistic and attainable. They should be aligned so they contribute to your overall well-being. Besides considering these factors, assign a deadline to your goals to track progress and for self-accountability. You can diversify your goals by setting short-term and long-term objectives as you progress. Short-term goals provide quick wins and motivation, while long-term goals help you maintain focus on sustained progress.

Regular Assessments

Regular assessments offer concrete data points that gauge your balance improvements. They help you understand trends and pinpoint areas requiring attention. Consider using standardized balance tests, like the Tandem Stand, where you stand with one foot in front of the other to test your balance duration. This test and several others were explained in the first chapter to let you understand your balance and body's limitations.

Perform assessments at regular intervals, every few weeks, to track changes and progress. Document the results of your assessments in your workout journal, noting the specific metrics. Transform assessments into enjoyable challenges by involving friends or family. Share your results and create a friendly competition to keep your motivation high.

Using Technology

Technology can be a powerful tool for tracking progress, offering data-driven insights and convenience. Explore fitness apps designed for tracking workouts. These apps often allow you to input exercise details, visualize progress through charts and graphs, and set reminders for your balance exercises. Consider using wearable devices like fitness trackers or smartwatches.

They track metrics such as step count, balance duration, and heart rate during exercises. Embrace the gaming aspect of fitness apps. Many apps offer rewards, achievements, or virtual badges for meeting goals, making tracking progress feel like an exciting game.

Consulting a Professional

Seeking guidance from a fitness or healthcare professional provides objective assessments and personalized advice for your balance exercises. Consider working with a physical therapist, personal trainer, or balance specialist with expertise in balance exercises. These professionals often have access to specialized equipment and tests to conduct thorough assessments. Collaborate with your fitness professional to set clear milestones and celebrate achievements together. Having a supportive partner can be motivating and enjoyable.

Revising and Updating Your Routine

Doing the same exercises every day can make your routine boring. Shuffle the stretches, warm-ups, and balance exercises daily to prevent stagnation and to keep your progress on track. You can review your workout journal to evaluate your progress, identify the areas you need to improve, and consider adding exercises for these areas when revising the exercise routine.

Introduce New Variations

Update your balance exercises by introducing new variations or increasing the difficulty. This keeps your routine fresh and engaging. Embrace the excitement of trying new exercises. Exploring fresh movements can reignite your passion for balance training, making the journey more enjoyable and rewarding.

Incorporating these strategies into your balanced exercise routine ensures on-time tracking of progress and adds depth and excitement to your fitness journey. Remember, it's not only about reaching your destination. It's about enjoying each step as you progress.

Gradually Increasing Difficulty

Over time, you will become more comfortable performing balance exercises as your muscles regain strength. Turn it up by increasing the difficulty level to reap maximum benefits. This approach enhances your balance abilities by putting it through challenging situations, reduces the risk of injury, and promotes muscle coordination. Before reading the how-to section for safely increasing the difficulty of your balance exercise routine, here's why stepping up the game is crucial to improving your balance and overall health.

Why Gradually Increase Difficulty?

Progression and Improvement

Slowly increasing the difficulty of your balance exercises ensures continuous progression and improvement in gait and balance. It allows you to build upon your abilities and challenge yourself to reach new milestones.

Preventing Plateaus

Your body can adapt and reach a plateau when you consistently perform the same balance exercises without increasing the difficulty. At this point, you might notice diminishing returns in improvements. Gradual progression helps you break through these plateaus and keep your balance exercise routine effective.

Injury Prevention

Pushing your balance exercises to become significantly harder too quickly can lead to overuse injuries or accidents. Gradual progression minimizes the risk of strains, sprains, or falls by allowing your body to adapt and develop the necessary strength and coordination.

How to Gradually Increase Difficulty

Incremental Changes

Start by making minor changes to your balance exercises. For example, if you're performing a static single-leg balance, aim to increase the duration by a few seconds each week. This gradual increase challenges your stability without overwhelming your body.

Add Variations

Introduce variations or modifications to your exercises. For instance, if you've mastered standing on one leg with your eyes open, progress to doing it with your eyes closed. This added sensory challenge requires heightened proprioception and balance.

Balance Games

You can include balance games in your exercise routine on alternate days to make balance training more engaging while increasing the difficulty through entertaining games. It might be difficult to play challenging exercises like the balance beam challenge, so it's better to replicate the game by creating a random path on the floor using chalk or removable colored tape. You must complete the path within a specific time without letting your feet move away from the path. To challenge yourself, create a random path each time to further refine your balance skills.

Integration with Other Skills

Besides adding exercises or increasing difficulty, combine your balance exercise routine with other activities you enjoy. For example, start your exercise routine with dancing, replacing warm-ups and stretching.

Multi-Planar Movements

Explore balance exercises involving movements in multiple planes. Movements like lateral lunges, diagonal reaches, or figure-eight patterns challenge your balance from various angles, enhancing overall stability. However, don't start these intense exercises before consulting your physiotherapist.

Balance Challenge Log

Create a log where you note down specific challenges you encountered during each exercise session. For instance, if you found it difficult to maintain balance while turning your head, jot down the details. This log can help you pinpoint areas for improvement.

Interval Training

Implement interval training into your balance exercises. Alternate between periods of high-intensity balance challenges and short rest intervals. Interval training can boost your cardiovascular fitness while increasing the intensity of your balance exercise routine.

Elevation Changes

Seek out changes in elevation for your exercises. Balance on different surfaces, like stairs or inclined planes, to create new balance challenges that mimic real-life situations.

Use Balance Props

Incorporate balance props into your routine. Tools like foam pads, balance boards, or resistance bands create instability, forcing your body to work harder to maintain balance. Start with less challenging props and gradually move to more advanced ones.

Complex Movements

Progress to more complex movements that involve dynamic balance. For example, walking on uneven surfaces like grass or sand, stepping over obstacles, or moving your arms while balancing on one leg. These dynamic exercises simulate real-life scenarios and enhance your functional balance.

Increase Sets and Repetitions

Gradually increase the number of sets or repetitions for each exercise. This elevates the overall workload and promotes strength and stability gains. For instance, if you started with two sets of 10 repetitions, progress to three sets of 15 repetitions.

Consult a Professional

Consider consulting a fitness trainer or physical therapist if you need more clarification about progressing safely. They can assess your current abilities, tailor your balance exercises to your specific needs, and guide suitable progressions based on your goals and limitations.

Listen to Your Body

Always pay close attention to how your body responds to the increased difficulty. If you experience pain, discomfort, or excessive fatigue, scaling back or modifying your exercises is crucial. Overexertion can lead to injuries, so prioritizing safety is essential.

Remember, patience is critical when gradually increasing the difficulty of your balance exercises. It's a process that takes time, and there's no rush to reach advanced levels. By systematically and safely challenging your balance abilities, you'll reap the benefits of improved stability, reduced fall risk, and enhanced overall physical well-being.

Overcoming Plateaus in Balance Exercises

Understanding Plateaus

A plateau in fitness is when you experience a halt or a significant slowdown in your progress. In balance exercises, a plateau means you're no longer seeing improvements in your stability, coordination, or overall balance despite consistent efforts.

Why Plateaus Occur

Adaptation

Your body is highly adaptive. When you perform the same exercises repeatedly without changes, it becomes more efficient at those movements, making it harder to challenge your balance.

Lack of Variation

If your exercise routine lacks variety, your muscles and nervous system might not receive the diverse stimuli needed for continued growth.

Overtraining

Excessive training without sufficient rest and recovery can lead to plateaus or even a decline in performance due to accumulated fatigue.

Nutrition and Hydration

Inadequate nutrition and hydration can affect your body's ability to recover and perform optimally, potentially leading to plateaus.

Stress and Sleep

High stress and inadequate sleep can hinder your body's ability to adapt and improve.

Strategies for Overcoming Plateaus

Change Your Routine

The most common cause of plateaus is sticking to the same exercises. Introduce new balance exercises or variations to break through. For example, if you've mastered single-leg stands, try single-leg stands on an unstable surface or add arm movements to challenge your stability.

Increase Intensity

Gradually increase the intensity of your exercises. You can do this by extending the duration of each exercise, increasing the number of repetitions, or incorporating more challenging props like balance discs or wobble boards.

Deload Weeks

Integrate deload weeks into your training schedule. During these weeks, reduce the intensity and volume of your balance exercises to allow your body to recover fully. Deloading can help break through plateaus by giving your muscles and nervous system a chance to reset.

Mental Imagery

Engage in mental imagery exercises where you vividly imagine yourself successfully performing challenging balance tasks. Studies have shown that mental rehearsal can positively impact physical performance.

Alter Recovery Strategies

Reevaluate your post-exercise recovery routine. Incorporate techniques such as foam rolling, stretching, and self-massage to alleviate muscle tension and improve circulation, which can aid in overcoming plateaus.

Vary the Environment

Change the environment where you perform your balance exercises. It could mean practicing outdoors on uneven terrain or different flooring, introducing a fresh set of challenges for your balance.

Cross-Training

Engage in cross-training activities that complement your balance exercises. Strength training, flexibility work, and cardiovascular exercises contribute to better overall balance.

Periodization

Implement a periodization plan for your training. Periodization involves organizing your workouts into phases, each targeting specific goals. It helps prevent overtraining and promotes steady progress.

Proper Nutrition and Hydration

Ensure you're consuming a balanced diet and staying hydrated. Nutrients and fluids are vital in muscle recovery and performance. If you don't focus on your nutrition, you might not see progress and increase your chances of injury.

Stress Management

Practice stress management techniques like meditation, deep breathing, or yoga. High stress negatively impacts your ability to make progress.

Adequate Rest

Allow your body to rest and recover between intense balance exercise sessions. Overtraining can hinder progress and increase the risk of injury. Besides overtraining, never push your body to its limits, as these exercises don't require putting the muscles or your body under stress.

Sleep

Prioritize quality sleep. Sleep is when your body undergoes repair and recovery, making it essential for physical improvements.

Consult a Professional

If you consistently face plateaus despite your best efforts, consider consulting a fitness trainer or physical therapist. They can provide expert guidance, assess your routine, and offer personalized strategies to overcome plateaus.

Monitoring Progress

As discussed earlier, keep meticulous records of your balance exercises. Regularly assess your balance abilities to track subtle improvements and identify plateaus. Remember, plateaus are a natural part of the fitness journey, and with patience, determination, and strategic adjustments, you can overcome them and continue progressing in your balance exercises.

Mindful Self-Assessment

Beyond physical metrics, practicing mindfulness during your balance exercises will provide valuable insights. Pay attention to how you feel mentally and emotionally during each session. Are you more confident? Less anxious about losing balance? These intangible improvements are as important as the physical ones.

Balance Metrics

While balance exercises often involve subjective assessments, consider incorporating objective metrics into your tracking process. Tools like force plates or wearable sensors provide precise data on your balance performance, offering a quantitative dimension to your progress tracking.

Functional Assessments

Progress in balance exercises should translate into improved functional abilities in daily life. Keep a log of practical improvements, like your ability to walk on uneven terrain without stumbling or reaching for objects on high shelves with greater ease.

Video Recordings

Recording your balance exercises on video can be a valuable tool for self-assessment. Reviewing your movements allows you to identify areas of weakness or imbalance that may not be apparent during the exercise. It also helps you refine your technique.

Setting SMART Goals

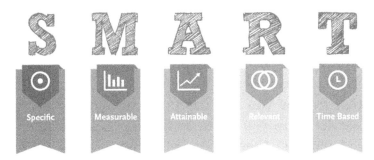

Specific

Specify the exact aspects of your balance exercises you want to improve. For instance, if you're working on single-leg balance, set a specific goal like "increase single-leg balance duration to 60 seconds."

Measurable

Ensure your goals are quantifiable. Use metrics like time, repetitions, or distance to track your progress. For example, you can measure your progress in seconds, inches, or repetitions.

Achievable

Goals should be realistic and attainable. Consider your current abilities, and avoid setting objectives too ambitious or unattainable in the short term.

Relevant

Align your balance exercise goals with your broader fitness and health objectives. Ensure they contribute to your overall well-being.

Time-Bound

Set a timeframe within which you intend to achieve your goals. A deadline creates a sense of urgency and keeps you focused.

The Role of Patience

Understanding Plateaus

Plateaus are a natural part of the fitness journey. Recognize that progress may not always be linear, and it's okay to experience periods of slower improvement.

Consistency

Consistency is key to overcoming plateaus. Continue your balance exercises even during plateau phases, as consistent effort often leads to breakthroughs.

Positive Reinforcement

Celebrate your successes, no matter how small they may seem. Acknowledging your achievements boosts motivation and helps maintain a positive attitude, even during challenging times.

Adapt and Adjust

If you encounter a prolonged plateau, don't be afraid to adapt your routine or seek guidance from a fitness professional. They can provide fresh insights and strategies to help you progress.

Long-Term Perspective

Keep the long-term perspective in mind. Balancing progress in balance exercises with overall health and well-being ensures you're not only chasing short-term gains but also maintaining a lifelong commitment to your fitness.

By incorporating these additional elements into your tracking and goal-setting process, you create a holistic approach to monitoring your progress in balance exercises. This comprehensive strategy enhances your understanding of your fitness journey and empowers you to make more informed decisions for continued improvement.

Chapter 8: Staying Safe

In this exhilarating journey toward improved balance and mobility, safely doing balance exercises is paramount. Besides being determined and knowing the proper instructions, understanding how to exercise safely prevents the body from potential strains, sprains, or injuries. This chapter shares valuable information about common exercise mistakes most seniors make, practical tips to protect you from injuries, and highlights the necessity of consulting healthcare professionals.

When doing balance exercises, improper form, not following instructions, overtraining, neglecting warm-ups, and several other blunders lead to pitfalls in your fitness journey. These frequent mistakes result in injuries, acting as an adversary in your quest to keep your gait balanced and the body healthy. Understanding these mistakes and implementing adequate safety protocols protects you from exercise-related injuries. The chapter is divided into three sections. In the first section, common balance exercise mistakes are shared, providing valuable insights into these blunders.

The second section explains practical tips and strategies to protect you from injuries. Thirdly, the necessity of contacting healthcare professionals will be discussed, as some people can't do balance exercises due to persistent medical conditions, diseases, or mobility issues. Without further ado, here are the most common balance exercise mistakes made by seniors.

Common Exercise Mistakes to Avoid

Skipping Warm-Up

The most common mistake many seniors make is skipping their warm-up routine before the exercise and starting immediately. Warm-ups before exercise are essential as they slowly increase the heart rate, raise body temperature, and prep the muscles and blood flow throughout the body. Proper warm-ups prime the joints for exercise, reduce stiffness, and mitigate the risk of muscle strains.

Similarly, slowly cooling down decreases the heart rate and reduces the build-up of lactic acid in the muscles, which causes muscle cramps. A cool-down routine after exercise also boosts body restoration and reduces stress.

Before starting your balance workout, spend at least five to ten minutes performing a light aerobic activity like brisk walking or stretching the muscles. Likewise, after the workout, you can do yoga or static stretches to relax the muscle groups used during the exercises.

Improper Footwear

Wearing improper footwear will only increase the risk of ankle sprains, limit ankle mobility, destabilize balance, and even result in falls while performing balance exercises. For example, wearing high heels, worn-out shoes, or other footwear that causes instability is a big no. Several feasible options include athletic shoes, shoes with non-slip soles, and custom footwear to provide stability, increase ankle mobility, and have good arch support.

Overestimating Abilities

Rushing into complex balance exercises can lead to falls, frustration, and potential injuries, especially if you haven't built a solid stability foundation. Start with basic balance exercises, like single-leg stands or heel-to-toe walking. As you gain confidence and strength, progressively challenge yourself with more advanced exercises.

Poor Posture and Form

Incorrect posture can strain muscles, cause joint misalignment, and compromise the effectiveness of balance exercises. Focus on maintaining proper alignment and posture. Keep your spine neutral, engage your core, and avoid excessive leaning or slouching. Seek guidance from a fitness professional if you're unsure about your form.

Holding Your Breath

Holding your breath can increase blood pressure, cause muscle tension, and hinder your ability to stay relaxed and focused during exercises. Breathe naturally and rhythmically throughout your exercises. Coordinate your breath with your movements, exhaling during the most challenging part of the exercise and inhaling during the less demanding phase.

Ignoring Progression

Your balance gains may plateau without progressing, and your workouts become less effective. Gradually increase the difficulty of your balance exercises. For instance, adding instability (e.g., using a balance pad), increasing duration or repetitions, or incorporating more challenging variations.

Not Using Support

Using support is entirely acceptable, especially if you're a beginner or have balance issues. Avoiding support when needed can lead to falls and discourage you from continuing with balance training. It's better to use support when necessary and gradually reduce your reliance on it as your balance improves. Safety should always come first.

Ignoring Pain or Discomfort

Pain is your body's way of signaling that something is wrong. Ignoring it can lead to injury or exacerbation of an existing issue. If you experience pain during a balance exercise, stop immediately and assess the cause. Consult a healthcare professional or physical therapist to address the issue before resuming the exercise.

Lack of Focus

Being distracted or not fully concentrating during balance exercises could cause instability and an increased risk of falls. Always perform these exercises with focused attention.

Ignoring Asymmetry

Neglecting to address the balance and stability needs of both sides of your body includes not balancing exercises that work one leg or side of the body as effectively as the other. Our bodies are not perfectly symmetrical, and favoring one side will cause imbalances in strength and stability, affecting overall balance and increasing the risk of falls. Incorporate exercises that target each side of your body equally. For example, if you do single-leg stands or leg lifts, make sure to perform them on both legs to maintain balance and symmetry.

Improper Progression Timing

Advancing to more challenging balance exercises too quickly without first mastering the foundational exercises. Rushing progression elevates frustration, decreases confidence, and increases the risk of falling, as you may not have developed the necessary stability and skill. Focus on mastering simpler balance exercises before attempting more complex ones. This gradual progression ensures you build a solid foundation and are better prepared for advanced challenges.

Overreliance on External Support

Leaning heavily on walls, handrails, or other external supports during balance exercises to the extent that you rely on them for stability. Excessive dependence on external support hinders the development of your intrinsic balance and core stability. Using support for safety is essential. However, reduce your reliance on it as you become more comfortable with balance exercises. Gradually decrease the support to challenge your balance progressively.

Neglecting Core Engagement

Failing to engage the core muscles effectively during balance exercises will cause instability and poor balance control. A strong core is the foundation of balance and stability. Without core engagement, your body will struggle to maintain equilibrium during exercises. Make a conscious effort to activate your core muscles during balance exercises. Focus on drawing in your abdominal muscles and maintaining a stable core to improve balance and control.

Improper Head Position

Holding your head in an unnatural or fixed position, for instance, looking down at your feet or tilting your head excessively during exercises. Head positioning is vital in balance. Improper alignment will cause neck strain, affecting overall stability. Keep your head neutral, looking straight ahead during balance exercises. This promotes proper spinal alignment and reduces unnecessary neck and upper back tension.

Inadequate Recovery

Not allowing sufficient time for recovery between balance exercises or workout sessions results in fatigue, decreased performance, and an increased risk of falls, as tired muscles are less responsive and coordinated. Incorporate rest periods between balance exercises and workouts to allow your muscles and nervous system to recover. Rest intervals provide the energy and focus for subsequent exercises.

Rushing through Exercises

A common mistake is performing balance exercises too quickly or with jerky, uncontrolled movements, rather than deliberate, controlled motions. Rapid or uncontrolled movements disrupt your balance and coordination, increasing the risk of falls or injuries. Execute balance exercises with slow, controlled movements, emphasizing proper form and stability throughout each repetition. Focus on quality over quantity.

Skipping Dynamic Balance

Concentrating exclusively on static balance exercises and neglecting dynamic balance challenges that mimic real-world movements develops bad habits. Dynamic balance is crucial for daily activities and preventing falls. Ignoring it can lead to instability in situations requiring movement. Include exercises that involve movement to improve dynamic balance and adaptability, like walking on uneven surfaces, stepping over obstacles, or shifting your weight while balancing.

Not Adapting to Age-Related Changes

Failing to acknowledge and adapt your balance exercises for age-related changes in strength, flexibility, and mobility. Aging can bring physical changes, and ignoring these factors develops frustration or injury during exercises. Choose age-appropriate balance exercises and consider limitations or changes in your body's abilities as you age. Adapting exercises to your current condition ensures safer and more effective workouts.

Disregarding Feedback

Ignoring feedback from your body during balance exercises, like not adjusting your posture or movements when you feel unstable or uncomfortable, is detrimental to your journey. Your body provides valuable cues about your balance and stability. Disregarding these signals makes you susceptible to accidents or injuries. Be attentive to how your body responds during exercises. If you feel unsteady or experience discomfort, adjust the exercise or seek guidance to ensure safety and progress in your balance training.

Neglecting Progress Tracking

Not keeping a record of your balance progress makes it challenging to assess improvements or identify areas needing improvement. Maintain a workout journal to track your balance achievements and setbacks.

Overtraining

Excessive training without adequate rest causes fatigue and decreased balance performance. Balance exercises require recovery just like any exercise.

Poor Nutrition

A lack of proper nutrition impacts your energy levels and overall fitness, which affects your balance. Ensure you're fueling your body with a balanced diet.

Including balancing exercises in your workout regimen will improve your general physical health, coordination, and stability. Avoid these frequent blunders and prioritize safety, correct technique, and progressive advancement in your balance training to maximize the benefits while reducing the risks. See a physical therapist or fitness expert for advice on a customized program if you're new to balancing exercises or have special difficulties.

Practical Tips to Prevent Injuries

Start with a Stable Base

Initiating your balance exercise from a stable position means you begin in a posture where both feet are firmly planted on the ground. You can gradually shift your weight from this base and transition into the specific balance exercise. Starting with a stable base provides a strong foundation. It minimizes the risk of losing balance or wobbling as you shift your weight during the exercise. It is particularly crucial for seniors who may have balance challenges.

Use Support as Needed

When you're unsure of your stability or are new to balance exercises, having a stable surface nearby to hold onto for support lightly is advisable. This support could be a chair, countertop, or sturdy railing. Having a support structure readily available offers a safety net. It helps you maintain balance and boosts your confidence when performing balance exercises, reducing the risk of falls, especially if you're still building your balance skills.

Mindful Progression

Mindful progression means gradually increasing the intensity and complexity of your balance exercises. It involves adding more challenging movements or incorporating props like balance pads or stability balls as your confidence and proficiency grow. Progressing in a controlled and thoughtful manner ensures that your balance abilities develop safely. Rushing into advanced exercises will cause frustration and an increased risk of falls or injuries.

Proper Lighting

Ensure that the area where you're performing balance exercises has sufficient lighting. Good visibility helps you spot potential obstacles, hazards, or irregularities in the flooring. Insufficient or poor lighting invites missteps and accidents during balance exercises, particularly if you can't see potential tripping or slipping hazards.

Stay Hydrated

Drinking water before and after your balance exercise routine is crucial to maintaining proper hydration. Dehydration causes muscle cramps and dizziness, which interferes with your ability to maintain balance. Adequate hydration is essential for overall well-being. Dehydration can cause discomfort and impair your physical and mental performance, including your balance.

Well-Fitted Clothing

Wearing well-fitted, comfortable clothing that allows freedom of movement is vital when doing balance exercises. Avoid clothing that is too tight or restrictive. Proper attire ensures your clothing doesn't interfere with your balance or range of motion during exercises. Loose or restrictive clothing affects your comfort and balance.

Mindful Breathing

Paying attention to your breathing during balance exercises involves inhaling and exhaling rhythmically and naturally. This practice helps you stay calm and focused during the exercise. Proper breathing enhances your relaxation and concentration, aiding your ability to maintain balance while preventing dizziness or breath-holding, disrupting your performance.

Secure Exercise Area

Ensure that the area where you perform balance exercises is free of clutter, rugs, or slippery surfaces that pose a tripping or slipping hazard. A clear and unobstructed exercise space minimizes the risk of accidents. It allows you to focus solely on the exercise and reduces the chance of stumbling or falling.

Warm-Up Gradually

Warming up before balance exercises involves light, low-intensity activities or movements that prepare your muscles and joints for the challenges ahead. A gradual warm-up increases your heart rate, blood flow, and body temperature. This prepares your body for exercise, reduces the risk of muscle strains or stiffness, and ensures your muscles are ready for the demands of balance exercises.

Listen to Your Body

Pay close attention to any discomfort, pain, or significant fatigue you experience during balance exercises. If you encounter pain, it's essential to stop the exercise immediately and assess the cause. Pain is your body's way of signaling something may be wrong. Ignoring it can lead to injuries or worsen an existing issue. Understanding and respecting your body's signals is crucial for safe and effective exercise.

Regular Check-ins

Periodically consulting your healthcare provider or a physical therapist to assess your overall health and balance abilities is essential. They offer guidance, monitor your progress, and ensure your balance exercises are appropriate for your current condition. Regular check-ins ensure your balance exercises align with your health needs and goals. Your healthcare provider can help you make informed decisions about your exercise routine and overall well-being.

Stay Consistent

Incorporating balance exercises into your routine regularly is crucial. Consistency in your practice helps maintain and improve balance. Regular practice ensures your balance skills remain sharp and develop as you age. It also reinforces the neuromuscular adaptations necessary for maintaining stability and preventing falls.

By following these detailed injury prevention tips, seniors can safely and effectively perform balance exercises, reducing the risk of accidents and injuries while reaping the benefits of improved stability and overall well-being. Remember, safety and adaptability are key, and tailoring your balance exercises to your abilities and needs is essential.

Consulting a Healthcare Professional

Consulting with a healthcare professional, especially for seniors, is not only a recommendation but also often a necessity when embarking on a fitness journey that includes balance exercises. Here's an in-depth explanation of the necessity of consulting with a healthcare professional:

Customized Exercise Plans

Healthcare professionals, including physicians, physical therapists, and registered dietitians, can assess your specific health status, physical strength, and existing medical conditions to create a personalized exercise plan that suits your unique needs. Seniors often have varying fitness levels, underlying health issues, and physical limitations. A customized exercise plan ensures your balance exercises are safe and effective, considering your strengths and weaknesses.

Safety First

Healthcare professionals can identify potential risks or contraindications related to your health or medical history. They can guide you on exercises that will exacerbate certain conditions or those that could lead to injuries. Safety should be the top priority for seniors when engaging in physical activities, especially those involving balance. You can minimize the risk of accidents and adverse health events by consulting a healthcare professional.

Managing Chronic Conditions

For seniors with chronic conditions such as diabetes, hypertension, or osteoarthritis, healthcare professionals can recommend balance exercises to improve stability and help manage these conditions. Balancing exercises with chronic conditions requires careful consideration. Healthcare professionals can ensure your exercise plan aligns with your medical needs and contributes positively to your health.

Medication and Interaction Awareness

Healthcare professionals will review your medications and investigate potential interactions or side effects that might affect your ability to perform balance exercises. Some medicines impact balance, coordination, or blood pressure. A healthcare provider can make necessary adjustments or offer guidance to mitigate these effects during exercise.

Fall Risk Evaluation

Healthcare professionals assess your risk of falls based on factors like muscle weakness, gait abnormalities, or balance impairments.

Seniors are at an increased risk of falls, which can have severe consequences. Healthcare providers can identify and address specific risk factors, recommend appropriate exercises, and provide strategies for fall prevention.

Regular Monitoring

Periodic consultations with healthcare professionals allow ongoing monitoring of your health and progress. They can adjust your exercise plan to accommodate changes in your health or physical condition. Health conditions evolve. So, regular check-ins with healthcare providers ensure that your balance exercises align with your health status.

Motivation and Accountability

Healthcare professionals will motivate, encourage, and guide you, helping you stay committed to your balanced exercise routine. Maintaining a consistent exercise regimen can be challenging, especially for seniors. Having a healthcare professional as a source of support and accountability can boost your adherence to your fitness goals.

Holistic Approach

Healthcare professionals often approach senior well-being holistically, addressing physical fitness and factors like nutrition, mental health, and social support. Senior health is multifaceted, and addressing all aspects of well-being is essential for maintaining a high quality of life. Healthcare providers can offer guidance on various health-related issues, creating a well-rounded approach to balance exercises and overall health.

Consulting a healthcare professional is a necessity for seniors pursuing balance exercises. These professionals offer personalized guidance, prioritize safety, manage chronic conditions, ensure medication compatibility, assess fall risk, provide ongoing monitoring, offer motivation, and take a holistic approach to senior well-being. Their expertise helps seniors reap maximum benefits from balance exercises while minimizing potential risks, ultimately leading to a healthier and more fulfilling life in the golden years.

Chapter 9: Lifestyle Tips

Although the various exercises and balancing techniques in this book are helpful, their effectiveness can be vastly increased if coupled with the right lifestyle choices. Nutrition, sleep, and mental health awareness are all crucial aspects of wellness. Balance exercises have their place but can only get you to a certain point without additional lifestyle changes. Holistic change must be embraced to address the body as its unified expression. Certain dietary plans can directly influence your balance and support your ability to stand strong. As you engage your muscles and joints to stretch and balance, you should also be engineering your mind and the internal environment.

Regularly exercising is the easy part. The bulk of your commitment and discipline will be channeled into the other crucial steps to maintain your body. Developing a narrow-minded focus on health is easy, especially if you see some results. But a multifaceted approach to your well-being will elevate you beyond what you imagined. Your health is your true wealth, so directing your energy into your well-being will open up much more room to explore the wonders of life in your elderly years. Minor adjustments can have surprisingly big impacts, so you can gradually shift to life-changing health protocols. How you live your life and your habits are far more impactful than two sessions a week of strenuous exercise. Therefore, any balancing activities you do are only one finger on the hand of well-being.

Lifestyle choices are the difference between being bedridden, immobile, and constantly in the hospital or having time to enjoy with your family and friends. Exercising without making the appropriate changes in your diet, sleep, and stress management behaviors is robbing yourself. The choices you make in between your workouts will guide your success. Slowing down aging to stretch your productive years is possible if you have the drive to follow through. Take the first step toward living better by treating your mind and body with the love they deserve.

Nutrition for Balance

What you put in is what you get out. You cannot throw sand into a fuel tank and expect the car to drive smoothly. This sort of abuse is what many people do to their bodies. A healthy diet can drastically impact a multitude of age-related health issues. Nutrition should be a pressing concern for the elderly because it changes your metabolism. Age brings physical transformations that will certainly impact the quality of your life. As people age, many experience a decrease in appetite caused by numerous reasons, like sensory impairment or diminishing gastrointestinal and oral health.

Since many older people are not getting their daily nutritional requirements through food due to eating less, many diseases can follow. Two illnesses linked to nutritional deficits affecting your balance are sarcopenia and osteoporosis. Sarcopenia is the loss of muscle that comes with age. Osteoporosis is when your bones become brittle. Many elderly people develop anorexia (NB: not anorexia nervosa which is a mental health issue) due to malnutrition caused by eating too little. Therefore, you must make sure the food you eat packs a nutrient-dense punch, and you supplement everything you are not getting.

Your skeleton is your structural support, bolstered by your muscles. Your nerves help you gather physical sensations, allowing you to determine how to respond to external stimuli. The combination of your bones, muscles, and nervous system is vital to your balance. The lack of vitamin D can contribute to brittle bones and cause muscular deterioration, increasing the probability of sustaining a harmful fall. Calcium helps promote healthy bones, while vitamin B12 helps repair damaged nerves. Since you may not be getting all these nutrients because of your changing eating patterns and gut health that come with age, you should consider taking supplements. Consult your doctor before taking any product.

Chronic illnesses like diabetes, heart disease, and atherosclerosis become more prevalent with age. On top of these illnesses, there is the added adverse impact of polypharmacy, the combination of taking five or more pills. Combining many pills has an accumulation of side effects that may need to be treated by adding even more medication. If your nutrition is high it will decrease your risk of developing chronic illness, eliminating the need for polypharmaceutical interventions.

The typical view of human sensory perception being limited to five senses is an incomplete understanding of how people function. The vestibular system comprising various parts of the inner ear is an overlooked sense that works in tandem with visual, auditory, olfactory, and touch input to create the complex balancing process. Your nervous and vestibular systems, along with your senses, receive inputs, your brain processes the input, and your musculoskeletal system produces outputs. These systems involve several body parts. Therefore, an overall nutritional scheme supporting these interlocking parts is the best way to promote health.

Convenience has allowed many to replace good nutrition with easy food. Whole foods are the best option for overall health. Heavily processed foods have large amounts of sodium and sugar, which could be detrimental, especially when you get older. Healthy vegetables and fruit supplemented with lean meat and high-fiber whole grains create a balanced diet, ultimately assisting you with physical balance. The interconnectivity of the body means everything is linked, so adjustments to your eating habits must be made from the vantage point of the whole.

Do not think of your nutrition as a diet because that word may have negative connotations created by the media. Your nutrition is about giving your body the fuel to maximize its functionality. Therefore, dieting culture must be reframed as creating a more positive relationship with food. It is no secret that food that is bad for you usually tastes great, but you spend so little time of your life eating. Do not sacrifice living well for 90% of your existence for the couple of minutes you spend in front of a plate.

Planning is the name of the game for building a wholesome, healthy diet. Your meals should be carefully monitored to consume beneficial food. Spending time at night packing and preparing food for the next day is an amazing way of monitoring what you eat. Meal preparation is a nutritionist's dream because you can carefully craft foods that promote collagen production for flexibility and contain the appropriate vitamins and minerals for bones and muscles to function supremely well.

Limit carbohydrates and manage your protein intake to decrease your sugar and build muscles. Many nutrient-dense foods do not have many carbs. Processed foods have the worst carbohydrates at levels detrimental to maintaining a healthy body. Always read the label before purchasing anything to ensure the sugar content is low and the protein content is reasonably high. Plant proteins are preferable to an excess of animal protein, so mix up your diet by adding a little of everything. A good rule of thumb is to aim for fresh products instead of products packaged in plastic and tins.

Sleep and Balance

Sleep is one of the most underrated aspects of maintaining a healthy lifestyle. Having a good night's sleep is like a magic pill with overwhelmingly positive health outcomes. Not only does being well-rested promote better mental health and physical activity throughout the day, but it also reduces the risk of falling and hospitalization. Older people are lighter sleepers and often wake up during the night. Therefore, you must make sure to get the required hours of sleep your body demands, especially with the increased physical activity of exercise. A melatonin supplement can help you get higher-quality sleep if you experience restless nights.

Sleep specifically has an adverse impact on postural balance, maintaining your center of gravity. Therefore, if you plan to work on your balancing abilities, missing hours of sleep is a huge barrier to that goal. Sleeping enough could profoundly impact how well you can move unassisted. Furthermore, adjusting your sleeping patterns is a change that can be made immediately without much effort. Exercising and eating right need commitment. Sleeping requires merely stepping into your ability to have a well-deserved rest.

The body needs to work, and it needs to rest. The interplay between exerted energy and recovery is what helps build overall wellness. There are some challenges with getting a full night's sleep when you age. Elderly people require at least seven to nine hours of uninterrupted sleep. However, factors like pain, illness, and medication could keep a person up at night. This low-quality sleep causes an increased prevalence of falls, memory loss, and irritability. Therefore, the appropriate interventions must be explored so you can take charge of your sleep cycle.

You can embrace several techniques to improve the length and quality of your sleep so you can wake up fully rested. Firstly, you must stick to a regular sleep schedule. Going to bed and waking up at the same time every day allows your body to adjust to a habitual sleep cycle. If your bedtime is different every day, it causes irregularity that can result in interrupted sleep. Next, you should avoid napping in the late afternoon. Naps feel great in the moment, but they can keep you staring at the ceiling, regretting your decisions in the middle of the night.

What you eat and drink also affects sleep. Alcohol and caffeine are terrible twins for getting that evening's rest. Caffeine, especially when drunk later in the day, can be overly stimulating. Alcohol is a little more deceitful because it fools you into thinking that it helps you sleep. However, it greatly diminishes your ability to sleep through the night and almost guarantees you will constantly be waking up. Large meals before bed can cause discomfort when sleeping, so watch what you eat in the evenings. The best thing you can do is eat at least three to four hours before sleep to give yourself time to digest your food. Setting up an early dinner routine can make a world of difference for your well-being and is a relatively easy adjustment.

Controlling the room you sleep in is an essential component of good-quality sleep. Avoid looking at screens like cellphones or television at least two hours before bed. If you can, keep those devices out of your room. The temperature should be set neither too hot nor cold to ensure peak comfort. Also, setting the mood with dim lights in your bedroom can facilitate better sleep. Set up a bedtime routine, like taking care of your skin or participating in whatever you feel gets you ready for bed. A bedtime routine mentally prepares you by allowing you to physically slow down and get in the right frame of mind to rest.

Remaining consistent in your exercise routine will help you sleep better. The physical fatigue of working out will make you so tired you will easily drift away into dreamland. However, be careful not to exercise within the last three hours of your going to sleep because this could disturb your sleep cycle. Exercise gets your blood running, so you will be hyperstimulated right after a workout. The opposite of being hyper is needed for sleep, so instead, opt for calming activities like soft classical music or reading a book right before bed.

Over time, low-quality sleep caused by sleep apnea, insomnia, or waking up multiple times a night to use the bathroom accumulates. The impact of one night is already significant, so over the long term, it is extremely detrimental to your physical and mental health. Sleep is like a reset where your body gets the opportunity to put everything back in order, like a mini-maintenance. Similarly, if you neglect anything you own by avoiding maintenance, the effects of sleep deprivation will worsen over time, leading to depression, anxiety, diminished postural control, and an increased risk of chronic illness.

Your medication also affects your sleep. If you have been prescribed medication by your doctor or are taking over-the-counter medication, ask a professional what will work best with the drugs to increase your sleep quality. Doctors can develop and adjust the medication combinations to work well with your body for sleep and rest. Communication with your doctor will be welcomed because only you can inform medical professionals about the side effects your medication has on your sleep schedule. By becoming more proactive in the medicine you consume, you can direct your prescriptions according to your needs. Sometimes, people fall into the trap of not wanting to be a burden and simply sucking up issues that medication cause. But your well-being should not be perceived as imposing. Speaking to your general practitioner or family doctor will only give them more insight into your health, benefiting you in the long run.

Stress Reduction Techniques

Aging can be a very stressful time in a person's life. The bodily and mental changes are sometimes destabilizing. Stress is often referred to as the silent killer because it creeps up unnoticed and is normalized in modern society. The impacts of stress are amplified with age because symptoms like high blood pressure can lead to chronic heart diseases. Your mental well-being and physical health are intrinsically linked because an ailing body affects your mental state, and a stressed mind affects your physiology.

Surprisingly, stress affects your balance when you are moving and standing still because of the increase in cortisol, the primary hormone released during stressful periods. It can be difficult to pinpoint the causes of stress because so much in your environment can be triggering, from work to your social status and the realities of aging. Therefore, you need coping mechanisms for a variety of contexts. The rat race has made sure that people are accustomed to constantly being under stress. The impacts of the consistent tension stress causes can be ignored in your younger years, but the effects become more apparent as they pile up. Therefore, you must find ways to open that internal valve and let off some of that stressful steam.

Your age shows resilience, which is the ability to respond to stressful situations. Now, all you have to do is find ways to bolster that resilience and introduce some novel coping strategies. The first step to combating stress is to introspect and discuss what causes your stress with someone you trust. Consciously exploring what causes you mental anguish puts you in a better position to address it effectively. You do not want to be a burden to others, so, understandably, you keep your stresses bottled up. But suppressing your emotions does not serve your well-being.

Once you have identified your stresses, you can implement interventions when they occur. Meditation and the Eastern practice of Qi Gong are healthy activities that reduce stress. Slowing your breathing and movements while being present in the moment releases the antioxidants in your body to aid in relaxation, bringing all the benefits of combating stress. The slight hormonal differences become more significant as you age, so stress can turn into something deadly. Participating in relaxing activities is, therefore, life-saving.

You can incorporate Qi Gong and yoga exercises into your balance work regimen. You are already adopting a regular workout schedule, so fuse a relaxation protocol with your strenuous physical activity. Working out is already a stress reliever, so combining it with the calm, calculated movements of Qi Gong or the breathing and stretching of yoga could create a mindfulness session that elevates you to the next level of wellness.

Touch is another stress-relieving activity that can be implemented anywhere. A relaxing massage done on yourself or by a partner can release stored-up tension in the body. Give yourself a deep tissue neck rub or massage your temples in a circular motion when you feel pressure building up. A loving touch from yourself or others can instantly bring down your cortisol levels and get you back into a calm, peaceful state that is fertile soil for health. Ask a loved one to help you out with a little shoulder rub or dig into your neck when sitting and watching TV. Even a two-minute massage daily can make a difference. Do not underestimate the power of touch because not much can compete with a gentle, loving massage to melt the stress off your body.

Spend time with loved ones and take up recreational hobbies to take your mind off your life stressors. Nothing is quite like a good distraction to get your mind in order. Overthinking, worrying, and stress are tied at the hip, so getting out of your mind with a bit of fun is highly recommended. Do what you enjoy doing and allow yourself to let go. The freedom grown from being carefree occasionally will translate into your workouts. Moreover, the enjoyment of life gives you a reason to be healthy. It will keep you on track and motivated to push forward with your physical activity and nutritional planning.

Dealing with your stress can prevent other mental issues from developing down the line. General population genetics are an indicator of proclivity to clinical depression, but with age, stress becomes one of the main ways to predict the development of depression. Therefore, cutting stress off at the root will help build sustainable mental wellness. Depression in your later years can leave you unable to embrace the fullness of existence in its unfiltered form. Dealing with your stress using conscious breathing and recreation is the equivalent of removing the blurry goggles that dim the technicolor of aging. The intersection between your mental and physical health becomes increasingly important as you age. Falling into a depressive state can quickly cause many ailments to flare up, which begins an endless cycle of deterioration mentally, emotionally, and physically. As soon as you notice the signs of psychological distress developing, it is of the utmost importance to address them immediately.

Journaling can be a valuable tool for reducing stress because it allows you to slow down and process your thoughts. Aging can be a rapid transformation in an individual's later years, so it makes sense that many are adversely impacted mentally by the reality of getting older. However, when you take time to sift through your concerns and face them head-on, the weight will be lifted off your shoulders. Recreation, meditation, and Eastern practices catered to inducing relaxed states, like gentle yoga or Qi Qong, filtered through awakened introspection, are the perfect cure for stress.

Chapter 10: Real-Life Success Stories

Reading about these balance exercises and stability-enhancing regimes may have got you all pumped up, but when you hop on the mat to start exercising, do you find it hard to muster the strength for even warming up? You might think that balance training is probably not for you. Remove that thought from your mind right away. Losing the desire to work out, being unable to gather the strength, and experiencing sudden lethargy are common responses during the initial stages, not only among seniors but also in younger people.

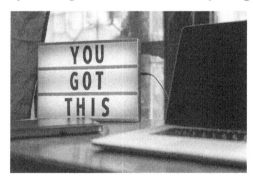

51. All you need is a little push on the first day, a little less on the second, and less still on the third until balance exercises become a habit. Source: https://www.pexels.com/photo/black-and-white-laptop-2740956/

All you need is a little push on the first day, a little less on the second, and less still on the third until balance exercises become a habit. Without a doubt, they will eventually become an integral part of your routine. There is no better way to push yourself to take that first step than reading inspiring real-life success stories.

Phyllis' Unique Journey

There was a time when Phyllis could hardly walk without losing her balance. Her posture was ill-defined, primarily because she had mild scoliosis. Completing a single push-up (with her knees on the ground) was impossible, and her flexibility was akin to an iron rod.

Phyllis began her journey of regaining her balance and strength with a few mild exercises with a trainer. It didn't take long for her to reach the moderate level, surpassing the one push-up mark. As her exercises slowly increased in intensity, her push-up count reached a more than satisfactory level (10 push-ups). She can stand on one leg for a little less than three minutes. She can even hold a hundred-pound weight in her hands with barely a strain.

Furthermore, she can hold a plank for more than two minutes (many younger people can barely hold it for a minute). Her daily workout routine has allowed her to regain her posture and prevent her scoliosis from worsening. Moreover, she is four times more flexible than before, almost as supple as a willow twig, and is as healthy as any person over 50 can be.

Phyllis doesn't consider her workouts as routine exercises. She says it is a way to understand and interact with her body. This unique viewpoint of socializing with herself has enabled her to develop a healthy relationship with her body. Each exercise acts as fodder for its growth. Since she started her balance and strength journey, she believes her confidence has scaled to new heights, especially while indulging in her favorite hobby, dancing.

Smiling All the Way

Have you ever seen anyone smile while working out? Most people are either grimacing under strain or wincing in pain. Not Beverly, an active, cheerful senior who is always smiling while exercising. Her face lights up with a full, warm smile, especially while performing her favorite workout, barbell curls. However, she wasn't always so chipper.

A few years ago, someone very close to her passed away. She couldn't move on from the loss, which affected her work and health. She is an online teacher, but during her distressing period, she rarely scheduled lectures due to her deteriorating health. Over time, she became so frail that she couldn't even climb the stairs to her apartment. It was around this time that she began her strength and balance training.

Determined to transform her health, Beverly performed her exercises with full vigor. Sometime during her training, she began loving certain workouts and started smiling while doing them. It was probably the first time she had given a heartfelt smile since her mourning period. The happiness at finally moving on, combined with her dedication to the workout routine, made her hale and hearty within under five months.

Today, she can walk up the stairs without support and even perform weighted exercises on the climb. Her balance has improved tenfold since she can maintain a tandem stance (heel-to-toe position) for more than two minutes. Her thirst for more challenging exercises remains unquenched, as she keeps smiling to build a healthy and balanced posture.

Beverly is grateful to her trainer for teaching the exercises and motivating her to keep going. But her trainer credits her cheerful attitude for the rapid improvements in her health.

An Inspiring Tale of an 82-Year-Old Youth

Once upon a time, Elizabeth (82 years of age) couldn't get a good night's sleep. The nagging pain in her hands would wake her up at odd hours. Additionally, her awkward posture and dwindling stamina caused her to pass her waking hours steeped in unease. She had a passion for traveling, which was snuffed out because of her inability to walk for long. Concerned about her deteriorating health, she took up strength and balance training courses.

Her journey to refuel her strength and reclaim her lost stamina wasn't easy, but working out under the watchful eye of a trainer twice a week helped her achieve her goals. After about one year, the hand pains that kept her awake vanished, never to return. She can get a full seven to nine hours of uninterrupted sleep. Her energy is off the charts for someone her age, and her posture has regained symmetry. Walking is no longer a problem since her stamina has improved in leaps and bounds.

She achieved benefits other than her goals, which were a pleasant surprise. The proportion of her waist and hips is not unlike that of a supermodel, and her flexibility can almost be compared to a novice gymnast. Do you want to meet Elizabeth to congratulate her on her spectacular transformation? Get in line because she is busy traveling around Asia, probably walking across a picturesque landscape and feeling proud of her achievements.

The Fight Against Parkinson's

Parkinson's disease attacks your central nervous system, as it slowly but surely affects your entire body, leading to complete loss of movement. There is no cure. Just one hope. Balance and flexibility exercises. Jennie Goodwin, a Parkinson's patient, fervently latched onto that hope.

She hired a Pilates instructor who focused on improving her balance and flexibility. Jennie was given a daily workout routine, which she undertook with enthusiasm. In only two months, the rigidity in her muscles and bones reduced considerably. Her overall body structure stabilized, and she no longer needed a crutch to walk upright.

She stresses that as her posture became more refined, her confidence and belief in herself also increased. She is still afflicted with Parkinson's, but it's not as severe as before. The symptoms have significantly abated, so much so that she doesn't feel the weight of the disease as she goes about her day.

A Daughter's Love

Ian's pride lay in his ability to walk upright, which many people his age couldn't do. It was shattered when he suffered a stroke. As his fitness decreased, he started drooping more and more while walking until he couldn't stand erect. He had to use a cane to stand, but no matter how hard he tried, he couldn't straighten his spine. His head was always hanging low, not only out of a bent posture but also from shame. It affected his physical health and mental well-being.

His daughter couldn't stand to watch him spiral down a path filled with dark thoughts. So, she decided to give him the tools to pull himself back up. Hiring Ian a fitness trainer, ensured all his problems and goals were addressed. Ian was skeptical at first, but as the training sessions progressed, he realized he didn't need to live with a bent posture, and his hope shone brighter.

He performed all the strength and stability workouts as instructed at least three times a week with complete dedication. Over time, his posture made a significant improvement. Five years of having a bent posture was corrected in less than five months. It was a magnificent display of strength training benefits. He can walk straight with his head held high for a few minutes. It's enough of an inspiration for him to keep pushing himself further.

Ian says that he is always fatigued after every training session, but the good kind of fatigue makes him feel like a new man. His daughter's unconditional love has paid off because he is always happy and smiling these days as he slowly regains his lost pride for walking upright.

Joseph's Pre- and Post-Pandemic Story

A 74-year-old man who had maintained his fitness most of his life had to suddenly undergo treatment for cholesterol and high blood pressure problems 13 years ago. That was the day his health worsened each year. His name is Joseph Agostino, and he had a weak posture with hip problems and dire weight issues.

There was a time when Joseph practiced ballroom dancing regularly (the secret to his once prolonged excellent health). However, since his treatment and medications left him with a poor posture, he couldn't continue dancing. After a few years, when his hip pains became unbearable, he decided to apply for a strength and posture correction program. He was excited to begin his training, but as luck would have it, the world was hit with the COVID-19 pandemic on that very day.

The program was postponed indefinitely, and Joseph had to live with his post-treatment problems while worrying about getting infected with the virus. It was a harrowing time for him. It took two long and excruciatingly painful years for his luck to change when the program was restarted in 2022. Throughout this tenure, Joseph kept his hopes alive and hit the ground running when his training finally began.

During the preparation period, he realized he not only had hip sciatica but was also afflicted with diastasis recti (a wide gap between the rectus abdominis muscles). However, it didn't get him down. He trained vigorously for three days a week and was committed to his homework during the other four days.

It took him no more than three months to experience life-changing improvements in his posture and flexibility. His hip movements have become more fluid, and his bodily afflictions have been reduced. Regularly performing balance and strength exercises have also subdued the pain. His hopes of making a full recovery are as high as ever, and his trainer believes it won't be long before the pain subsides completely.

The 90s Are the New 60s

People aged 90 and above often regret living for so long. They are known to reminisce about the early days of their seniority, the 60s and 70s, when they could enthusiastically tackle their problems. Then, thoughts about letting it all go and giving up on life haunt their heart and soul. But this is not the case with Jim, a man born in the Greatest Generation.

He has worked out in the gym for most of his life. Indoor exercises aside, he has also done bike trails and hikes from time to time. No wonder he didn't face major health problems in his senior years. However, soon after he entered his 90s, his balance began to falter while walking, and he would often stumble and fall. Over the course of a few months, he felt weaker and weaker, forcing him to quit cycling and hiking.

After seeking a professional opinion, he started doing balance exercises and took up strength training. The first few days of training were exhausting. Of course, most people his age probably wouldn't have been able to muster the strength to take those first steps. But Jim did, and his progress beyond those initial stages was rapid.

He trained with a group of seniors, many much younger than him. Needless to say, he proved a constant source of motivation for them. His raw energy and ardor for performing the exercises inspired everyone around him to do better. Today, he can walk for a long time without stumbling and has become much stronger than before. This sprightly nonagenarian is planning to resume cycling and hiking shortly.

Conclusion

Reclaiming your strength and courage doesn't have to be limited by age. You can start anytime. The sooner you begin working on your balance and stability, the better. Aim for three balance exercise sessions each week, lasting around 30 to 45 minutes. This simple commitment can significantly transform your life.

Imagine confidently walking into a room without worrying about falling or needing a walking aid. Picture yourself with a fit and healthy body because balance exercises target various muscle groups, offering a holistic approach to fitness. As you grow older, you'll have something others envy: impressive balance and stability.

Growing older doesn't have to equate to a decline in health. Staying active and incorporating regular physical activity into your life can lead to a longer, more fulfilling journey. What's equally great is that by consistently exercising and staying active, you're adding years to your life and life to your years.

Many people often hold misconceptions about exercise. They think they're too old or not strong enough to engage in physical activity. The reality is quite different. Exercise is like a fountain of youth for the mind and spirit. It helps protect you from illnesses and chronic diseases, maintains your weight, and keeps you steady on your feet as you age.

The great thing about balance exercises is that you can do them in the comfort of your own home. There's no need for an expensive gym membership. You only need to set aside time for these exercises, get an exercise mat for comfort, pick comfortable workout clothes, and find supportive shoes to get started.

Here's a straightforward plan to get you going:

- **Schedule Your Sessions:** Make time in your weekly routine for your balance exercises. Consistency is key, so aim for regular practice for the best results.

- **Get the Basics:** Grab an exercise mat to make your workouts more comfortable. Wear comfy workout clothes and choose shoes that provide good support and stability.

- **Start Slow:** If you're new to balance exercises, begin with the easier ones and work up to more challenging routines as you build confidence and strength.

- **Get Expert Advice:** If you've recently had surgery, are dealing with specific health issues, or have questions about which exercises are right for you, consult a doctor or physical therapist. They can give you personalized advice to ensure your safety and progress.

Remember, your journey toward better balance and stability is an ongoing process. With determination and commitment, you can reach a balance and stability level that will significantly improve your life. So, get ready to take those first steps towards a stronger, more confident you. Your future self will be grateful.

Share and encourage others to restore balance and stability in their lives by leaving a review.

References

14 strength & balance exercises for seniors. (2020, October 9). Lifeline. https://www.lifeline.ca/en/resources/14-exercises-for-seniors-to-improve-strength-and-balance/

8 core exercises for seniors (pictures included). (2022, February 28). Lifeline. https://www.lifeline.ca/en/resources/core-exercises-for-seniors/

8 stretching and balancing exercises for older adults. (n.d.). Virtua.org. https://www.virtua.org/articles/8-stretching-and-balancing-exercises-for-seniors

9 stretching exercises for seniors. (n.d.). Onemedical.com. https://www.onemedical.com/blog/exercise-fitness/stretching-exercises-for-seniors/

A good night's sleep. (n.d.). National Institute on Aging. https://www.nia.nih.gov/health/good-nights-sleep

Aging changes in sleep. (n.d.). Medlineplus.gov. https://medlineplus.gov/ency/article/004018.htm

Amestoy, M. E., D'Amico, D., & Fiocco, A. J. (2023). Neuroticism and stress in older adults: The buffering role of self-esteem. International Journal of Environmental Research and Public Health, 20(12), 6102. https://doi.org/10.3390/ijerph20126102

Baiera, V. (2021, August 4). Best mobility workout for seniors: Complete guide. Step2Health; Vince Baiera.

https://step2health.com/blogs/news/best-mobility-workout-for-seniors-2021-complete-guide

Baiera, V. (2022, March 24). Seated balance exercises for seniors: 5 moves to try. Step2Health; Vince Baiera. https://step2health.com/blogs/news/seated-balance-exercises-for-seniors-5-moves-to-try

Balance exercise for seniors and the elderly. (n.d.). Eldergym.com. https://eldergym.com/balance-exercise/

Balance exercises : NCHPAD - building inclusive communities. (n.d.). National Center on Health, Physical Activity and Disability (NCHPAD). https://www.nchpad.org/636/2603/Balance~Exercises

Balance. (n.d.). Harvard Health. https://www.health.harvard.edu/topics/balance

Bastin, A. (2018, August 1). Active male seniors: How to train smart and recover faster. Lifeline. https://www.lifeline.com/blog/train-smart-recover-fast-tips-for-active-senior-men/

Bedosky, L. (2022, April 22). The best core exercises for seniors. Get Healthy U | Chris Freytag; Get Healthy U. https://gethealthyu.com/best-core-exercises-for-seniors/

Belanger, K. (n.d.). Phyllis's success story. Improve balance and flexibility. Weight loss. Vintagefitness.Ca. https://www.vintagefitness.ca/blog/2023/08/04/phyllis-success-story

Best balance exercises for seniors. (n.d.). WebMD. https://www.webmd.com/healthy-aging/best-balance-exercises-for-seniors

Best dynamic stretches for older adults. (n.d.). WebMD. https://www.webmd.com/healthy-aging/9-best-dynamic-stretches-for-older-adults

Billowits, E. (n.d.-a). 82-year-old remarkable fitness journey. Fitness for seniors, Toronto. Vintagefitness.Ca. https://www.vintagefitness.ca/blog/2023/06/23/success-story-82-years-old-improves-strength%2c-balance-and-endurance

Billowits, E. (n.d.-b). Fitness for seniors, success story. Balance and mobility. Vintagefitness.Ca. https://www.vintagefitness.ca/blog/2023/05/26/beverly-has-improved-her-balance-and-strength-with-exercise

Billowits, E. (n.d.-c). Success story. Posture improving. Fitness for seniors. Toronto. Vintagefitness.Ca. https://www.vintagefitness.ca/blog/2023/04/28/ian-has-improved-his-posture-and-feels-more-confident

Biswas, C. (2021, November 29). 10 core exercises for seniors to improve their stability. STYLECRAZE. https://www.stylecraze.com/articles/core-exercises-for-seniors/

Çay, M. (2017). The effect of cortisol level increasing due to stress in healthy young individuals on dynamic and static balance scores. Northern Clinics of Istanbul, 5(4), 295. https://doi.org/10.14744/nci.2017.42103

CDC. (2023, July 6). How much physical activity do older adults need? Centers for Disease Control and Prevention. https://www.cdc.gov/physicalactivity/basics/older_adults/index.htm

Choowanthanapakorn, M., Seangpraw, K., & Ong-artborirak, P. (2021). Effect of stress management training for the elderly in rural northern Thailand. The Open Public Health Journal, 14(1), 62–70. https://doi.org/10.2174/1874944502114010062

Churchill, R., Teo, K., Kervin, L., Riadi, I., & Cosco, T. D. (2022). Exercise interventions for stress reduction in older adult populations: a systematic review of randomized controlled trials. Health Psychology and Behavioral Medicine, 10(1), 913–934. https://doi.org/10.1080/21642850.2022.2125874

Commodari, E., & Di Nuovo, S. (2019). Perception of stress in aging: the role of environmental variables and appraisal of the life experiences on psychological stress. Neurology, Psychiatry, and Brain Research, 34, 28–33. https://doi.org/10.1016/j.npbr.2019.09.001

Cristina, N. M., & Lucia, D. (2021). Nutrition and healthy aging: Prevention and treatment of gastrointestinal diseases. Nutrients, 13(12), 4337. https://doi.org/10.3390/nu13124337

Cronkleton, E. (2020, May 11). Balance exercises for seniors: 11 moves to try. Healthline. https://www.healthline.com/health/exercise-fitness/balance-exercises-for-seniors

Cronkleton, E. (2020, May 11). Balance exercises for seniors: 11 moves to try. Healthline. https://www.healthline.com/health/exercise-fitness/balance-exercises-for-seniors

Dzierzewski, J. M., & Dautovich, N. D. (2018). Who cares about sleep in older adults? Clinical Gerontologist, 41(2), 109–112. https://doi.org/10.1080/07317115.2017.1421870

Eating Well - balance & dizziness Canada. (2019, July 5). Balance & Dizziness Canada - Supporting, Inspiring and Educating Those Affected by Balance and Dizziness Disorders; Balance & Dizziness Canada. https://balanceanddizziness.org/help-yourself/eating-well/

Etudo, M. (2022, October 10). Balance exercises for seniors: How to do them safely. Medicalnewstoday.com. https://www.medicalnewstoday.com/articles/balance-exercises-for-seniors

Findley, D. (2023, February 17). Warm-up exercises for seniors or over 50 • [video and guide]. Over Fifty and Fit; Dane Findley. https://overfiftyandfit.com/warm-up-exercises-seniors/

Freutel, N. (2016, January 13). Stretching exercises for seniors: Improve mobility. Healthline. https://www.healthline.com/health/senior-health/stretching-exercises

Functional Training. (2023, August 31). How can you avoid common mistakes and myths when training for balance? Linkedin.com; www.linkedin.com. https://www.linkedin.com/advice/0/how-can-you-avoid-common-mistakes-myths-when

Golden, N. (n.d.). Core exercises for seniors: Training the core for older populations. Nasm.org. https://blog.nasm.org/core-training-for-seniors

Gonzalez, J. C. (2021, September 14). 21 exercise equipment for seniors – how to choose the best one for your condition. Best Used

Gym Equipment.
https://www.bestusedgymequipment.com/exercise-equipment-for-seniors/

Good question: What's the Difference Between Stretching and Warming Up? (n.d.). Hospital for Special Surgery. https://www.hss.edu/pediatrics-difference-between-stretching-warming-up.asp

GoodRx - error. (n.d.). Goodrx.com. https://www.goodrx.com/health-topic/senior-health/balance-exercises-for-seniors

Hall, T. (2023, September 15). Crafting a balance routine: Personalizing stability workouts for clients. ASFA. https://www.americansportandfitness.com/blogs/fitness-blog/crafting-a-balance-routine-personalizing-stability-workouts-for-clients

Halvarsson, A., Dohrn, I.-M., & Ståhle, A. (2015). Taking balance training for older adults one step further: the rationale for and a description of a proven balance training programme. Clinical Rehabilitation, 29(5), 417–425. https://doi.org/10.1177/0269215514546770

Hernández-Guillén, D., Tolsada-Velasco, C., Roig-Casasús, S., Costa-Moreno, E., Borja-de-Fuentes, I., & Blasco, J.-M. (2021). Association ankle function and balance in community-dwelling older adults. PloS One, 16(3), e0247885. https://doi.org/10.1371/journal.pone.0247885

Hoesch, G. (2023, September 24). 8 tips for overcoming fitness plateaus. National Personal Training Institute Florida. https://nptiflorida.edu/8-tips-for-overcoming-fitness-plateaus/

Iwasaki, S., & Yamasoba, T. (2015). Dizziness and imbalance in the elderly: Age-related decline in the vestibular system. Aging and Disease, 6(1), 38. https://doi.org/10.14336/ad.2014.0128

Kaur, D., Rasane, P., Singh, J., Kaur, S., Kumar, V., Mahato, D. K., Dey, A., Dhawan, K., & Kumar, S. (2019). Nutritional interventions for elderly and considerations for the development of geriatric foods. Current Aging Science, 12(1), 15–27. https://doi.org/10.2174/1874609812666190521110548

Kutcher, M. (2021, February 1). Effective warm up for seniors (standing) — more life health - seniors health & fitness. More Life Health - Seniors Health & Fitness. https://morelifehealth.com/articles/standing-warm-up-routine-for-seniors

Kutcher, M. (2022, May 26). The complete guide to great balance for seniors. More Life Health - Seniors Health & Fitness. https://morelifehealth.com/articles/balance-guide

Langhammer, B., Bergland, A., & Rydwik, E. (2018). The importance of physical activity exercise among older people. BioMed Research International, 2018, 1–3. https://doi.org/10.1155/2018/7856823

LCMC Health. (2021, December 15). 6 tips for exercising safely as an older adult. LCMC Health. https://www.lcmchealth.org/touro/blog/2021/december/6-tips-for-exercising-safely-as-an-older-adult/

Lindberg, S. (2020, March 10). Chair exercises for seniors. Healthline. https://www.healthline.com/health/chair-exercises-for-seniors

Marcin, A. (2017, July 12). Ankle stretches: Strengthening, flexibility, and more. Healthline. https://www.healthline.com/health/fitness-exercise/ankle-stretches

Michiel, L. (2020, April 1). Building a home gym for seniors. Lori Michiel Fitness, Inc. https://lorimichielfitness.com/building-a-home-gym-for-seniors/

Ortiz, D. (2020, August 5). 7 causes of balance issues in the golden years. Home Care Assistance of Jefferson County. https://www.homecareassistancejeffersonco.com/what-can-be-causing-my-elderly-parents-balance-difficulties/

Savoie, L. (2021, June 28). Safety tips during balancing exercises. Ann's Professional Home Care. http://www.aphcinfo.com/safety-tips-during-balancing-exercises

Senior Fitness Tips and the mistakes to avoid. (2014, January 20). My Senior Health Plan. https://www.myseniorhealthplan.com/blog/2014/01/20/senior-fitness-mistakes-to-avoid/

Set, S. F. (2022). 13 best stretches for seniors that can be done standing or seated. SET FOR SET. https://www.setforset.com/blogs/news/stretches-for-seniors

Sites, S. (2022, December 26). 7 knee strengthening exercises for the elderly to try. Discovery Village; Discovery Village Senior Living. https://www.discoveryvillages.com/senior-living-blog/7-knee-strengthening-exercises-for-the-elderly-to-try/

Stelter, G. (2016, January 21). Tai Chi for seniors — 3 moves to improve balance and stability. Healthline. https://www.healthline.com/health/senior-health/ta-chi

Stone, K. L., & Xiao, Q. (2018). Impact of poor sleep on physical and mental health in older women. Sleep Medicine Clinics, 13(3), 457–465. https://doi.org/10.1016/j.jsmc.2018.04.012

Success stories. (2019, March 18). Balanceyourwellbeing.co.uk/wellbeing-journal/. https://www.balanceyourwellbeing.co.uk/success-stories/

The best core exercises for older adults. (2021, April 1). Harvard Health. https://www.health.harvard.edu/staying-healthy/the-best-core-exercises-for-older-adults

The importance of tracking your Fitness progress. (n.d.). Asirecreation.org. https://asirecreation.org/recreport/special-feature/592-the-importance-of-tracking-your-fitness-progress

The national council on aging. (n.d.). Ncoa.org. https://www.ncoa.org/article/5-tips-to-help-older-adults-stay-motivated-to-exercise

The national council on aging. (n.d.). Ncoa.org. https://www.ncoa.org/article/what-is-a-physical-therapist-and-how-can-physical-therapy-help-me

Tunturi. (n.d.). Tunturi New Fitness B.V. https://www.tunturi.com/en/blogs/blogs/the-benefits-of-an-aerobic-step/

Umemura, G. S., Furtado, F., Santos, F. C. dos, Gonçalves, B. da S. B., & Forner-Cordero, A. (2022). Is balance control affected by sleep deprivation? A systematic review of the impact of sleep on the control

of balance. Frontiers in Neuroscience, 16.
https://doi.org/10.3389/fnins.2022.779086

Usa, H. (2019, December 13). 5 types of balance and strength training equipment every senior fitness center should consider. HUR USA - FOR LIFELONG STRENGTH; HUR USA. https://hurusa.com/5-types-of-balance-and-strength-training-equipment-every-senior-fitness-center-should-consider/

Vanner, C. (2020, August 26). Fitness mistakes most seniors make. ActiveBeat - Your Daily Dose of Health Headlines. https://activebeat.com/your-health/senior/fitness-mistakes-most-seniors-make/

Varghese, D., Ishida, C., & Koya, H. H. (2022). Polypharmacy. StatPearls Publishing.

Yoga for seniors: Benefits, poses, chair yoga. (2021, February 8). Lifeline. https://www.lifeline.ca/en/resources/yoga-for-seniors/

Zapater-Fajarí, M., Crespo-Sanmiguel, I., Pulopulos, M. M., Hidalgo, V., & Salvador, A. (2021). Resilience and psychobiological response to stress in older people: The mediating role of coping strategies. Frontiers in Aging Neuroscience, 13. https://doi.org/10.3389/fnagi.2021.632141

Made in the USA
Las Vegas, NV
30 January 2024

85082416R00105